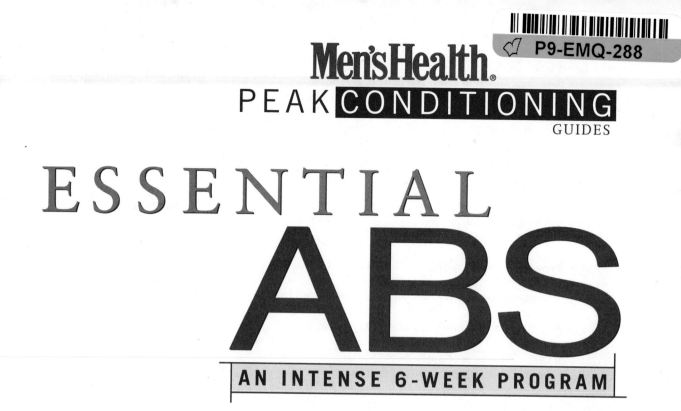

# Men's Health®
## PEAK CONDITIONING GUIDES

# ESSENTIAL
# ABS

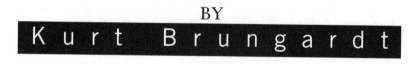

## AN INTENSE 6-WEEK PROGRAM

BY

Kurt Brungardt

RODALE

**Notice**

The information in this book is meant to supplement, not replace, proper exercise training. All forms of exercise pose some inherent risks. The editors and publisher advise readers to take full responsibility for their safety and know their limits. Before practicing the exercises in this book, be sure that your equipment is well-maintained, and do not take risks beyond your level of experience, aptitude, training, and fitness. The exercise and dietary programs in this book are not intended as a substitute for any exercise routine or treatment or dietary regimen that may have been prescribed by your doctor. As with all exercise and dietary programs, you should get your doctor's approval before beginning.

Interior and Cover Designer: Susan P. Eugster
Interior and Cover Photographer: Mitch Mandel/Rodale Images

**Library of Congress Cataloging-in-Publication Data**

Brungardt, Kurt, 1964-
    Essential abs : an intense 6-week program / by Kurt Brungardt.
        p.    cm—(The men's health peak conditioning guides)
    Includes index.
    ISBN 1-57954-292-1 paperback
    1. Exercise.  2. Abdomen—Muscles.  I. Title.  II. Series.
  GV508 .B79  2001
  613.7'1—dc21                   00-012331

**Distributed to the book trade by St. Martin's Press**

  4  6  8  10  9  7  5       paperback

Visit us on the Web at www.menshealthbooks.com, or call us toll-free at (800) 848-4735.

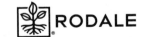

WE **INSPIRE** AND **ENABLE** PEOPLE TO IMPROVE
THEIR LIVES AND THE WORLD AROUND THEM

# CONTENTS

# INTRODUCTION

It's not easy being a guy these days. We're told we should have every element of the good life: a challenging, high-paying job; a knockout sex life; family and friends; plus time to relax and enjoy it all. And yet, at the same time, we want to have perfect bodies too.

Something's got to give. After all, unless that job pays so well that you can afford to change the Earth's rotational axis, there will never be more than 24 hours in a day.

And if that job is truly challenging, it's probably pretty stressful too. Stress increases your body's production of a hormone called cortisol, which causes fat to be stored in your midsection. Look around, and you'll see that most guys who get the great jobs have given up on the idea of having great bodies. And a lot of guys who have great bodies have given up on the idea of having great jobs—their bodies become their work.

But you don't have to make either of those compromises. It's possible to be successful in your career without being a pot-bellied member of the Future Myocardial Infarctions of America, a guy who can't get on an airplane without the flight attendant casting a nervous glance toward the defibrillator. And you don't have to give up the leisure time, the family and friends, or the explosive sex life. In fact, the better your body gets, the more combustible your sex life could become.

So what does all this happily-ever-after stuff have to do

with your abs? Just this: If you want the abs, you have to live the life. You have to do the things in this book, you have to do them intensely, and you have to do them consistently.

This book will ease you into a 6-week Core Program of abdominal exercise, aerobics, and careful eating. From there, you can go in any direction you want—stomp on the accelerator and become a full-fledged fitness animal, stay with the 3-hours-a-week Core Program, or find ways to get the same work done in even less time. Once you see how simple and enjoyable a balanced fitness program can be, I think you'll stick with it, in some form, for the rest of your life.

If you're in pretty good shape already, you may actually get cover-model abs by the time you finish the Core Program. But this book isn't written for the guy who's just 6 weeks away from his appearance in a bikini-underwear ad. It's for the rest of us, who look at those models and wonder, "How do I get there from here? How do I go from zero to six-pack?"

This book will show you how. It won't happen fast, it won't happen without effort, but the Core Program that author Kurt Brungardt has designed will show you the steadiest, straightest path there is.

Kurt knows that the most intimidating step is the first one—he's spent 18 years as a fitness trainer, along with all the health writing he's done. That's why this book is an introduction to fitness in general as well as to getting your midsection muscles to look their best.

Kurt and I have enjoyed all the benefits of being fit and healthy, and more than anything, we want you to find out what you've been missing. To us, this is the good life, and we don't want to keep it to ourselves.

—**Lou Schuler**
FITNESS EDITOR
*MEN'S HEALTH* MAGAZINE

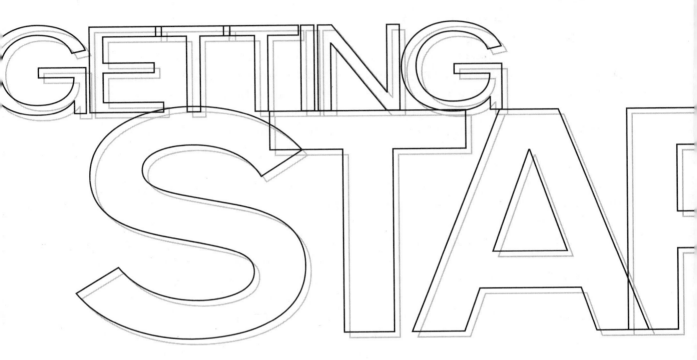

GETTING STARTED

RTED

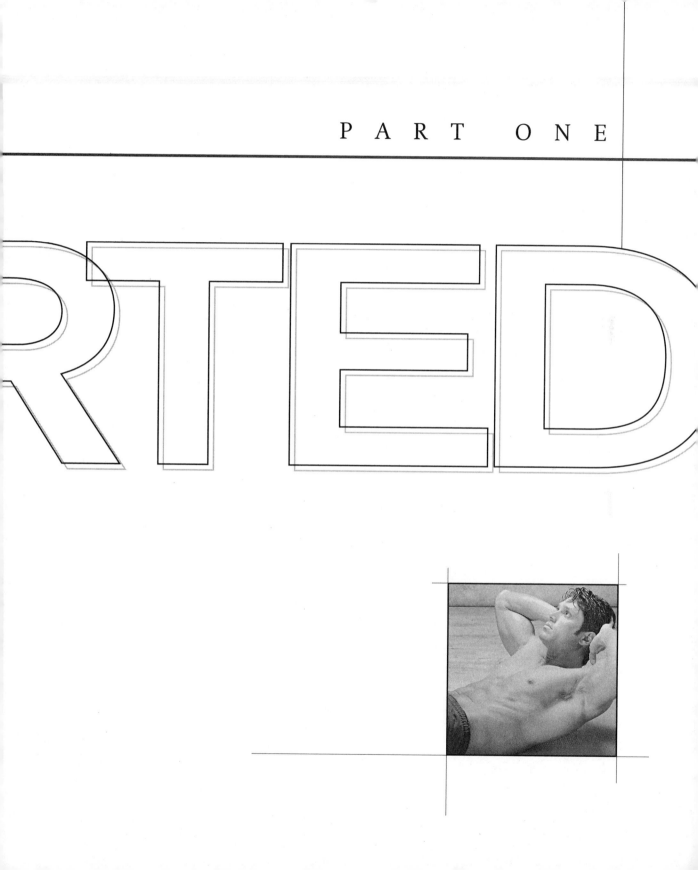

# ESSENTIAL ABS PLAN

Think of this book as your road map to Buff City. You know the place: It's where the flab that currently protrudes over your belt is nowhere to be found. It's where your abdomen is all grade-A muscle, with more definition than a dictionary. In Buff City, you literally stand taller, with better posture, thanks to your strong abs. There's less strain on your lower back, so it's easier for you to do everyday stuff like picking up boxes off the floor and wrestling your kid into his car seat. Your clothes fit better in Buff City—but the women there may want you to take them off more often. With *Essential Abs* as your guide, you'll soon be on your way to that destination, to the body you've always wanted.

You've heard the old saying "A journey of a thousand miles begins with a single step"? Never mind that today a 1,000-mile journey starts with a call to your travel agent or a visit to a discount-ticket Web site—the wisdom of the adage still holds true. But on your 1,000-mile trip to Buff City, you can easily take a 2,000-mile detour if your first step is in the wrong direction.

Magazines feature new ab workouts every month, TV ads offer quick-fix fitness products, and store shelves are stocked with "super" supplements for rescuing your troubled middle. This overdose of information has led to confusion about what truly is the best path to well-defined abdominal muscles.

The goal of *Essential Abs* is to get you started in the right direction and on the most direct route. Its philosophy is back to basics. This book will give you a solid foundation of knowledge and proven techniques for training your abs. No gimmicks, no gadgets, no miracles. Just results. You'll learn the fundamentals of exercise and nutrition. You'll establish exercise habits that you can build on throughout your life.

In 6 weeks, you'll progress from a modest 3 to 5 minutes of exercise a day to a robust 3 hours a week. You'll start with four simple midsection exercises—three for your abdominals, one for your lower back—and build on that base until you're doing a sophisticated series of abdominal exercises and three aerobic workouts a week. Plus, you'll be carefully monitoring your diet to ensure that you enjoy the full benefits of this new exercise habit.

## WHO IS THIS BOOK FOR?

This book wasn't written with the needs of the competitive bodybuilder in mind. It addresses three particular types of guys.

**The beginner.** He's thought about exercise, talked about exercise, maybe even bought a miracle belly-reducing nutritional supplement or a piece of infomercial exercise equipment. But he's never actually established an exercise habit.

**The active man.** *Essential Abs* is not for couch potatoes only. It's also for the guy who is active and energetic but who has never found a structured exercise program that works for him. Maybe he fig-

ured that he didn't have time to fit exercise into his busy schedule. Or maybe he never felt that he needed an exercise routine—until he noticed his metabolism slowing, his waist expanding, or the years of 8-hour, deskbound workdays taking their toll on his lower back.

**The frustrated-and-confused man.** Finally, *Essential Abs* was also written with a third guy in mind, the one who's been working out for a while—or, more accurately, trying to work out. But he's fallen into a vicious cycle of trying and failing, starting and stopping, with a net effect of either no results or, worse, a steadily declining physique and fitness level.

## WHAT YOU'LL LEARN FROM THIS BOOK

If you're one of those three guys, here's what *Essential Abs* has for you.

■ Basic abdominal anatomy
■ Proper technique for the most effective abdominal exercises
■ Planning strategies and goal-setting techniques
■ Motivational tips to help you harness the power of your mind
■ A progressive week-by-week program
■ A stretching routine that's ab-specific
■ A cardiovascular-fitness program
■ Nutritional advice to help you cut calories and see the results of your hard work
■ Lower-back exercises, which you'll do in tandem with the ab exercises

to create a protective sheath of muscle for your entire midsection
■ Advanced routines

This book is broken down into four basic parts. Part one will dispel the myths and the rumors about miracle cures and help you find a deep and sustaining motivation for staying on a fitness program. Part two will teach you principles and techniques for safe and effective abdominal training. Part three will guide you through the Core Program, a progressive ab-and-fitness regimen designed to promote wellness and trim and tone your abs. And part four will show you where to go from there to maintain your abdominal gains and improve your overall fitness.

The best course of action is to read the first two parts before starting the Core Program. If you're dying to get started, you can begin the Core Program and read the other chapters as you go. But it's very important to read all the chapters. They all contain essential information for achieving your goals.

## THE ESSENTIAL TRUTH

Ernest Hemingway said, "The best reason for telling the truth is because it's the easiest thing to remember."

That's why *Essential Abs* takes the easy way out by telling you that there is no fast track from a soft middle to rock-hard, beach-ready, six-pack abs. But there is a slow-but-steady way, and that's what this book offers.

Stick with *Essential Abs*, and it will stick with you. The Core Program gives you an exercise platform you can use for the rest of your life. You can build on it when you're ready for more challenging exercise routines or return to the very beginning when you need to cut back to a minimum.

That six-pack will come when you build enough muscle and lose enough fat. You're not guaranteed to achieve it in the 6 weeks that the Core Program covers. But you won't achieve it at all if you don't get started on a solid exercise program with a sensible diet.

So let's get going.

# 2

# ESSENTIAL FACTS

A pound of fat contains 3,500 calories.

A Big Mac contains 570 calories.

Doing 20 crunches burns about 9 calories.

In other words, a few minutes of abdominal exercise isn't going to make much of a dent in a lifetime's worth of accumulated fat. And one poor dietary choice—we picked on the Big Mac here, but it could be anything from a hot dog at the ballpark to pizza and beer at the Friday-night poker game—can undo weeks of targeted ab workouts.

I say that not to scare you off but to make sure that you understand the facts of abdominal exercise. And the first fact is that the exercises you do to build midsection muscles won't have much effect on the fat that surrounds them.

Hopefully, you already knew that, but every new infomercial product on the market seems to fly on the wings of a hope that people either don't know or are willing to forget this simple rule.

## AB CULTURE

A sculpted midsection has been the idealized epitome of masculine strength and attractiveness throughout history. The ancient Greeks and Romans depicted it in their statues of gods and godlike athletes and emperors. During the Renaissance, Michelangelo endowed his statue of David with a torso that is literally chiseled. A more recent incarnation appeared in the 1990s, in the ripped form of Marky Mark in those Calvin Klein underwear ads. Today, muscles in general and abs in particular are undoubtedly a status symbol. Washboard abs are everywhere: in health club commercials, in action movies, and on magazine covers.

The idea has become fixed in men's minds that not only is the perfectly chiseled midsection something to aspire to, but that there is a population of guys out there who have such a thing and who are ready to use it to take our women and—who knows?—maybe our houses, cars, and 401(k) funds too.

Ab guys have become to men what necktie-thin models are to women: an impossible ideal. Guys crowd into gyms, buy ab rollers, hire personal trainers, and continue to make the supplement industry a multibillion-dollar money-making machine, all with the idea that they're one exercise, cable machine, or protein shake away from the riches that life would bring if they had toned abs.

But what nobody ever sees is the truth about the physical icons with ripped abdomens. So here's the truth.

- Ab models are genetically gifted. If they weren't, they wouldn't be models in the first place (or at least not models who actually make a living at it).
- It's their job to be in perfect shape. They couldn't come into your office and crunch numbers the way you do, and you shouldn't expect to be able to step in front of a camera and crunch abs the way they do.
- You see them only on their very best days. Nobody stays shredded year-round.
- In the days before a photo shoot, models consume an unhealthy high-protein, low-carbohydrate diet.
- They often use drugs like ephedrine and caffeine to speed up their metabolisms and melt off the last bits of fat around their middles. And that's just for starters. Amphetamines, diuretics, steroids, growth hormones—name any muscle-building, fat-burning, or water-draining drug, and somebody in a commercial or on a billboard has taken it.
- Photography and filmmaking are all about illusion. Tricks of posing and lighting can work wonders. And sometimes the photos are touched up. Computers make it easier than ever to alter images.
- And don't forget, these models are holding their breath and flexing.

## NATURE VERSUS FASHION

Enough about ab guys. Let's talk about you.

As a man, you're predisposed to store fat in your midsection. It shows up there first and often lingers long after all the other fat on your body has been burned off.

This is why guys sometimes get disillusioned when they go on weight-loss programs and feel as if they've lost more off their faces than off their bellies. Guys whose cheeks are so hollow that they look like they just survived 6 months in a terrorist prison camp might still have love handles.

The other half of the equation is even more cruel: When you regain a few pounds, the first place they establish a beachhead is your belly.

But the news isn't all bad. First, nature has a plan when it stores fat in your midsection. It's not putting it there just to humble you at the beach. Fat is stored energy. It's what your body uses to get you through lean times. Your body wants you to use this fat. Our distant ancestors used

## ONE BAD APPLE SHAPE

If you put fat cells under the microscope, they all end up looking about the same, regardless of whether they come from your midsection, thigh, or big toe. But your body uses them differently, depending on where they're stored.

Men tend to accumulate fat in their upper bodies, mostly around their abdomens but also in their chests. This is called visceral or truncal fat, and it contributes to the dreaded apple shape. (The opposite is the pear shape, an accumulation of fat in the thighs and buttocks that's more common in women.)

Abdominal fat is very active metabolically; that is, it's there for sustained energy when you need it. In fact, you probably have enough stored energy in your fat cells to walk from Boston to Atlanta. With a few pit stops at Denny's, you could probably make it to Miami. Your muscles and liver, by contrast, contain enough sugar-based energy for only a 6- to 7-mile jog.

But when this ab fat sits on your body, unused, you pay a steep price. Abdominal obesity is highly correlated with Syndrome X, a series of deadly health problems that include high blood pressure and elevated levels of insulin, blood sugar, and cholesterol. The bottom line is that high levels of midsection fat are associated with diabetes, heart disease, and stroke.

How do you know if your level of visceral fat is high? Calculate your waist-hip ratio. Measure your waist at its narrowest point, probably around your belly button. Then measure your hips at their widest point. Divide your waist size by your hip size. Men with waist-hip ratios higher than 1.0 have double the death rates of men with ratios below 0.85. Men with ratios above 0.98 have 2.3 times the stroke risk of men who fall below 0.89.

But an even simpler measure of your risk is waist size itself. If it's over 40, that's trouble. If it's over 46, that's big trouble. So keep this in mind on those days when you're tempted to can your ab workout in favor of sitting around on your can.

their fat to carry them hundreds of miles in search of a woolly mammoth that would let them get within spear-throwing distance.

Women, by comparison, tend to store fat around their hips and thighs, and nature has an entirely different plan for it. The fat ensures that a fetus or nursing infant will have sustenance until the men return with the mammoth meat.

Once they've devoured that hairy pachyderm, nearly all men store fat preferentially in their middles, and we keep some of it there even when other areas of body fat have disappeared. But because abdominal fat is there to be used for energy, with enough work over a long enough period of time, most guys—including you—really can get rid of it.

## MYTHS AND FACTS

Though it is true that exercise can help you shed your abdominal fat and tone your abdominal muscles, there is a lot of false information out there about what types of exercise are most effective. Here are some of the most common misconceptions, along with the real deals.

**Myth:** Doing abdominal exercise will erase abdominal fat.

**Fact:** Spot reduction is physiologically impossible.

The beginning of this chapter already touched on this, but here's an example that helps illustrate the point. Picture a tennis player. If he's right-handed, his right forearm will have more muscle mass from hours of gripping and rotating his tennis racket. His other arm will be smaller and less defined, but it won't be fatter. Exercise burns fat systematically, according to patterns established by human anatomy and individual genetics. Targeting exercise to one region of the body or another won't make fat disappear off that particular region.

**Myth:** It takes hundreds of crunches to get ab muscles in shape.

**Fact:** Abdominal muscles are still muscles, and they don't respond to hundreds of repetitions any better than your biceps or chest muscles would. Just as you wouldn't do more than 15 repetitions in a set of biceps curls, so you shouldn't do any more than that for your abs.

When you can easily do 15 repetitions of any abdominal exercise, you need to either switch exercises or find some way to make that exercise harder on your muscles. Otherwise, you're just building endurance in the muscle, not size. And size is what makes a muscle look pumped, whether you're talking about biceps or abs.

**Myth:** Sports provide all the abdominal exercise anyone needs.

**Fact:** Targeted abdominal exercise can improve sports performance.

Chapter 13 gets into this in more detail, giving you a sports-specific abdominal routine. But for now, know that most sports certainly do place a great demand on your midsection, requiring strength, balance, and the ability to generate tremendous force. Training your ab muscles off the field will make it easier for them to do their job on the field.

Picture Mark McGwire playing first

base: He tightens his abdominals while waiting for the pitcher to throw the ball to the plate; this holds his body in a good position to move quickly if the batter hits the ball anywhere near him. Then, after the ball is hit to the shortstop, he might have to stretch his abdominals to catch an off-center throw and still get the runner out at first.

When McGwire steps up to bat, the muscles around his waist have to contract powerfully in a well-coordinated sequence with his legs, hips, shoulders, and arms so he can rotate his body hard enough to send the ball into the next zip code.

By strengthening and stretching these muscles in his workouts, Big Mac ensures that when he needs them they'll perform at the highest possible level. Remember that even the pros struggle with their middles. Two of the most common athletic injuries are lower-abdominal and lower-back strains.

**Myth:** Abs need to be trained every day.
**Fact:** Three times a week is the limit.

It's true that your abdominals are built more for endurance than for quick bursts of power. Their first job is to maintain your posture, which means they have to be ready to contract for hours at a time.

However, like all muscles, abdominals have a combination of fast- and slow-twitch fibers. It's the fast-twitch muscle fibers, the ones that make it possible to generate quick bursts of power, that have the most potential to grow. Those are the fibers you have to target when you do abdominal exercises.

After a workout, fast-twitchers need time to recover so they can come back bigger and stronger for the next workout. You should give them at least a day between exercise sessions to recuperate.

**Myth:** Abdominal exercise alone will produce great-looking abs.
**Fact:** It's possible, but adding aerobic exercise and a healthy eating plan will get you there faster.

Aerobic work is one of the best ways to burn calories, which you need to do to shed belly fat and expose the muscles underneath. You should also make sure that you eat a healthy diet so that you don't take in too many calories in the first place. Rock-hard abs won't impress anybody if they're buried under a layer of blubber.

# ESSENTIAL
# PEP TALK

I could talk all day about abdominal exercise, show you hundreds of exercises, and pass on dozens of programs and training tips. But it won't do you a bit of good if you don't stick with the program, if you exercise this month and then take next month off. You have to be consistent.

That's why I'm including motivational stuff in an exercise book. This chapter will give you strategies and techniques to help you set goals, deepen your commitment, and overcome the obstacles that you'll face on the journey.

## LOVING THE GAME

When you first start exercising, you view your body as an object, something outside yourself, something to be manipulated in a mechanical way. You do this exercise for that muscle, and hope you end up looking like the guy on the magazine cover.

But people who have been exercising for a long time—people who actually look forward to their workouts—connect to their bodies in a different way. They know how to use physical movement to create sensations they enjoy, from the opiate-like endorphin release that a distance athlete feels to the "pump" that a bodybuilder gets when his muscles are fully engorged with blood.

One guy might like the intense focus that's required to work out. Exercise can be a great escape after being bombarded all day by phone calls and e-mails and job-related crises. Another guy may enjoy the feeling of accomplishment and self-discipline that comes with exercising first thing in the morning, while the rest of the world sleeps.

Then there's the athlete, whose biggest thrill is competing, perhaps feeling his testosterone surge after methodically taking apart an opponent. The best illustration of this is Michael Jordan. Most athletes today sign contracts that limit the extracurricular sports activities in which they're permitted to participate. After all, if a player gets hurt in a pickup game, it's a multimillion-dollar loss for his team. But Jordan had a "love of the game" clause in his contract that allowed him to play basketball anytime and anywhere he wanted. Jordan needed to keep his competitive fires burning year round and was willing to risk injury rather than give up this sensation.

Whatever your game is, you know it's in your blood when *not* participating makes you feel bad.

But how do you get from your present sedentary state to an exercise high? After all, if you're reading this book, it's a good bet that you've never felt any particular connection to any physical activity. And when you've tried to get moving, you've felt much better after you've quit—the aches and pains of exertion go away, you return to eating the foods that make you feel happy and content, and you catch up on all the TV shows that you missed during your unfortunate forays to the gym.

Here are six strategies to help you get and stay motivated until your personal love-of-the-game clause kicks in.

## STRATEGY #1:
# SET GOALS

Motivation is directly linked to a plan of action. It's hard to get and stay motivated if you're not clear on where you're going and how you're going to get there.

Your goal should be specific and measurable. "I'm going to get buff" does not qualify. To turn this daydream into a goal, you need to define *buff*. Maybe what you really mean is that you'd like to lose 1½ inches off your waist. Write that down, put it in a place where you'll see it, and record your progress toward it.

For best results, establish short-term, intermediate, and long-term goals.

**Short-term goal:** In the case of the Core Program, such a goal is "I want to establish a consistent training regimen that includes ab exercises, cardio work, and healthful food choices."

**Intermediate goal:** "I want to get down to size 34 pants for my high school reunion next year." Measure your waist once a week and write down the result.

**Long-term goal:** "I want to look like this guy in the magazine." Cut out the picture. Tape it to your refrigerator or put it on the wall in your exercise area. Take pictures of yourself in the same pose every month or two, and watch yourself get closer to your ideal.

To achieve your short-term, intermediate, and long-term goals, you also need to set daily goals. You must take specific actions that are in line with your longer-range objectives. The operative word here is *specific*. Each day, set workout and diet goals.

- Make food choices that cut back your caloric intake. If you eliminate 500 calories a day, you'll lose about 1 pound per week.
- Know how many reps of each exercise you want to complete.
- Plan how many minutes of aerobic exercise you're going to do.
- Congratulate yourself when you achieve your daily goals.

This may sound a little excessive, but you need to be proactive. Read food labels and make smart choices. Push yourself during your workouts. Discipline yourself to keep an exercise journal—women love guys who keep journals.

Hey, if you wanted to lead a life of quiet desperation, you wouldn't have bought this book. Remember that each time you meet your daily goals, you set up camp a little bit closer to your big goals.

## STRATEGY #2:
# KNOW THE ENEMY

The name of your nemesis is homeostasis, which is your physiological system's urge to maintain the status quo. Your body will

## DROPPING THE LAME EXCUSES

Sometimes, your biggest barrier to having a great body is your state of mind. Before you can shed pounds, you may have to shed a self-defeating attitude. Some guys repeat patterns of behavior that are destructive, knowing deep down that they're sabotaging themselves but continuing anyway. They come up with seemingly logical excuses for giving up on their abs program.

Don't be one of those guys.

Here are some examples of common cop-outs and the responses you can use to call their bluffs.

COP-OUT: "How many muscles do I need to sit at a desk and type on a keyboard?"

REALITY CHECK: "Sitting at a desk all day is ruining my back. Doing abdominal and lower-back exercises will strengthen my back, improve my posture, and make my work more comfortable."

COP-OUT: "I'll get further in

life if I spend my time on my career instead of on my body."

REALITY CHECK: "These days, men are often judged by appearance as well as performance. If I'm out of shape, my boss may view me as undisciplined and a bad candidate for advancement."

COP-OUT: "I don't have enough energy for this."

REALITY CHECK: "Exercise will give me more energy in the long run."

resist change at the beginning of a fitness program, raising physical defenses against overexertion. It registers a sudden increase in exertion as a challenge to its energy reserves, hormonal balance, body temperature, blood sugar, and immune system. It will hold back many of its muscle fibers and nerve cells, limiting your strength. Your deconditioned cardiovascular system will make you feel winded and tired almost instantly. And for the first few days after exercise, you'll feel sore as hell.

The Core Program helps break down your physical defenses because it is designed to progress at a slow, gradual pace. This not only prevents injury but also prevents your body from rebelling.

## STRATEGY #3:
# FORGE PARTNERSHIPS

Friends and family can help or hurt when you're starting out. Your wife's initial encouragement of your self-improvement plan can quickly turn around. She might

## THE 11 COMMANDMENTS OF SELF-IMPROVEMENT

**1.** You must learn proper technique. **No matter what you're doing—abdominal exercises, tennis, weight lifting, whatever—learning to do it right is your first priority. This prevents injuries and ensures that you'll be successful in the long run.**

**2.** You must allow your body to recuperate. **This means giving it plenty of water and high-quality foods and as much sleep as it needs. Most guys need at least 7 hours of shut-eye a night, though some need as much as 9.**

**3.** You must continually challenge your body. **Your** body won't improve unless you give it progressively harder tasks.

**4.** You must exercise consistently. **That doesn't mean you should never take a break. But for the results you want, you need to stick with a program without taking extensive layoffs.**

**5.** You must believe that you can accomplish your goals. **If you don't, you will quit. If you do, you'll find a way to meet your own expectations.**

**6.** You must learn from your mistakes. **Most exercisers, at one time or another,** try to do too much and end up getting hurt. Or they pick an inappropriate program and find that the wrong things are growing while other things are shrinking. A mistake isn't a reason to quit, it's a chance to refine your goals and techniques.

**7.** You must reward yourself. **Exercise can turn into joyless monotony if you don't have a way to celebrate your successes. For a week or month of successful workouts, you could pick up a new CD or have dinner at a favorite restaurant. For losing 3 inches off your waist, you**

resent the time you spend away from her, feel threatened by your new self-control, or fear that when you stop being a schlump you'll immediately go trolling for a new, improved mate.

Friends might not want to lose a drinking buddy, a guy they can count on to join them for nachos and a couple of pitchers of suds during the Final Four.

Here are some ways to get everyone on your side.

**Encourage your wife or girlfriend to join you.** Even if she doesn't want to do the abdominal exercises, she might be up for a walk or bike ride.

**Offer reassurances.** If exercise involves time away from your family, try to make up for it later. If you go for a run on Sunday morning, do something special with your loved ones later in the day.

**Invite your buddies to your place for the game instead of going to a bar.** Have some lower-fat snacks available—even if you're the only one who eats them—and serve some light or even nonalcoholic beer.

**Find a training partner.** A workout buddy could buy yourself a new gas barbecue grill.

**8.** You must concentrate on the task. **If you stop in the middle of a set to answer the phone or you allow your children to disrupt your workouts or you watch TV between exercises, you're not allowing your mind to focus on the exercise. Without focus, you won't approach the exercises with any intensity, and without intensity you won't accomplish anything.**

**9.** You must keep an open mind. **It could be that great-looking abs aren't possible, given your genetics. Or per-haps your knees won't allow you to run as much as you need to in order to reach your goals. Your body always has some surprises in store for you. You can't anticipate them, but you can adjust your program and move on with new exercises and, perhaps, more realistic goals.**

**10.** You must be patient. **Sometimes results come fast but then taper off. Sometimes they come slow. Everyone gets frustrated with their pace of improvement. But you'll never know what your body is ca-pable of until you give it a chance to react to consistent exercise over a sustained pe-riod of time.**

**And, although it wrecks the biblical symmetry, here's the 11th commandment.**

**11.** You must not expect perfection. **Exercise is a process of giving your body new challenges and reveling in your new accomplishments. But you can't ever expect a moment when your body will be perfect. There will always be something new to work on. Look at your body as a lifelong project that will bring you much satisfaction as well as some frustrations. Enjoy each stage of the venture.**

can help you start and stick with a program. It makes you accountable to somebody—if you blow off a workout, you're not just hurting yourself, you're letting your partner down.

**Be a betting man.** If you're the competitive type, bet a friend or coworker that you can lose 10 pounds faster or drop 2 inches off your waist or finish a 10-K run or improve your bench press.

## STRATEGY #4:
# ACCEPT SETBACKS

Everyone gives in to an occasional indulgence or blows off a workout now and then. No one lives a perfect life. Here's how to deal with those little slipups.

**Plan them.** Some lifetime exercisers give themselves a weekly "cheat day" in which they can skip exercise and eat anything they want. If you're trying to lose weight, this could slow your progress since the calories you consume on a cheat day don't magically disappear. But you may enjoy the program more and stick with it longer if you know you can eat anything you want every Saturday.

**Get right back on the horse.** Say you go on a business trip and blow every part of your program for 4 days. You don't exercise, you overeat, you get sloppy drunk. You may feel that you have trashed all your progress. You haven't. Instead of saying, "Well, I screwed up. Guess I'll never be in shape," simply pick up where you left off. The longer you stick with your program, the faster your body will bounce back from these missteps.

## STRATEGY #5:
# OFFER YOURSELF LOTS OF VARIETY

There's a reason why an exercise program is often called a routine. It's a habit, something you do over and over again. But exercise isn't like brushing your teeth. You can't expect to do it the exact same way every time and get the results you want.

Athletes know this (or at least their trainers and coaches do), so they build variety into their training schedules. They might exercise at the same time almost every day, but they vary the exercises considerably. Sometimes they focus on strength, sometimes on developing muscle mass, sometimes on increasing speed, sometimes on agility.

Your training program can and should change regularly. Knowing you're going to do something different will get you more psyched up for a workout than knowing you're going to do the same old thing. That's why the *Essential Abs* Core Program is based on variety. You'll add new and challenging variables at each stage.

## STRATEGY #6:
# TAKE TIME OFF

Yeah, you're probably good at this one already. But, as hard as it is to believe, once a guy gets into a routine and starts seeing results, he can easily turn compulsive about exercise. While it was once a struggle to stick with a 3-days-a-week program, he might find himself exercising for weeks on end without taking a single day off.

Exercising too much can be a problem. Your body will break down if you don't give it time to recuperate. Even if you don't get compulsive, you still need to take breaks from a structured program.

Here are some ways take that break.

■ Always rest at least 1 day a week—do no formal exercise at all.

■ Never lift weights more than three times in a week if you're doing a total-body workout like the one in chapter 14. And always take at least 1 day off between workouts.

■ Every 6 to 8 weeks, rest for 1 full week. That means no goal-oriented exercise. You can still hike or take a bike ride or jog, but do nothing that involves a schedule, stopwatch, or training log.

# CHAPTER FOUR

# ESSENTIAL MINDSET

The number-one goal of *Essential Abs* is to teach you how to exercise—how to do specific abdominal moves, how to integrate ab exercises with aerobic work, and how to continue an exercise program so you create a healthy, vibrant, muscular physique of which you can be proud. To learn how to exercise, you need to train your mind as intensely as you train your body.

When an elite athlete integrates the power of his mind and the grace of his body, sportscasters say that he's "in the zone."

Another way to put that is to say that the athlete has achieved a flow state. This means that he's completely in the moment, completely unself-conscious, simply performing without stopping to judge his performance. You can learn to do this and make your workouts far more productive in the process.

## GOING WITH THE FLOW

In his book *Flow: The Psychology of Optimal Experience*, psychologist Mihaly Csikszentmihalyi outlines the elements that lead to a positive heightened experience that he calls flow. Csikszentmihalyi, a professor at the University of Chicago, interviewed hundreds of people from all walks of life: athletes, factory workers, the rich and powerful, and people who overcame extreme hardship. The goal of his research was to break down the elements that create flow experiences. Csikszentmihalyi's work shows that the richness and happiness of your life is determined by two things: one, where you choose to put your attention and, two, the quality of that attention.

You can increase the quality and enjoyment of your training sessions by consciously focusing your attention on the task at hand. Here are some of the key elements of flow as they relate to your ab training.

**Flow element 1: A challenging activity that requires skill.** A flow activity encompasses skills that can improve with practice. One of the keys to a successful exercise program is proper technique. Challenge yourself to go beyond just knowing the correct motion. The Core Program quickly takes you from the most basic movements to more complicated techniques. I didn't set it up this way to make you feel awkward and uncoordinated. I want you to force your body to learn complex, difficult moves. There is an art to doing ab exercises. Okay, ab work is not a masterpiece like a Reggie Miller jump shot or a Pete Sampras serve, but it's your sport, your event. Strive for the highest possible level of performance.

**Flow element 2: The merging of action and awareness.** If you want to achieve flow, you can't just zone out and do the activity. You have to pay full attention to what you're doing. This is challenging in ab work because your workouts aren't as exciting as a set of tennis or a basketball game, where there's an opponent and constant shifts in direction and momentum.

You have to look at this as an opportunity to practice the skill of focusing your attention.

You need to put your mind in your muscle when you train. This means putting 100 percent focus on the muscle you're training. If you're working your lower abs, give them 100 percent concentration. Feel your abs going through their range of motion and concentrate your mind on the task at hand. This tight focus increases your awareness of the movement, helping you isolate the muscles you want to work and minimizing the involvement of secondary muscles.

Each repetition and each workout must be filled with this level of quality. It may seem extreme, but the only guaranteed way to achieve a goal is by focusing your conscious mental and physical energy toward it.

**Flow element 3: Clear goals and feedback.** Flow requires that the activity be bounded by rules that clarify your goals and provide feedback. For example, in tennis you know that you've hit a good shot when the ball lands on the line and a bad shot when the ball flies out of bounds. The Core Program takes care of this element by giving you specific goals for each level.

**Flow element 4: Paradox of control.** Flow activities present variables that aren't completely under your control, even though you're functioning at a high level. For example, in a downhill ski run, the slope may be particularly challenging. In a tennis match, your opponent may just be at a higher skill level than you are. To apply this to your ab workout, give up your obsession with the results and just focus on the process. Accept the good and bad days, don't compare and despair, and strive to fulfill your potential. Give it your best shot, and understand that the results may be out of your control.

**Flow element 5: The loss of self-consciousness.** This means you let go of destructive self-criticism. Don't judge what you're doing while you're doing it. Stay in the moment of the task and complete it to the best of your abilities, without beating yourself up. If you miss a workout, don't get discouraged and view yourself as a failure. View it as a positive circumstance: You'll have more energy when you do your next workout.

Even when you combine all of these elements, flow is not an automatic response. You don't just start doing crunches and become magically transported into the zone. Professional athletes struggle with these elements from game to game, quarter to quarter, set to set, inning to inning. It's the same with you: Workout after workout, set after set, repetition after repetition, you'll work at getting better and more consistently finding the flow of your workouts.

## SEEING THE FUTURE

To achieve results, you must also be fully focused on your ultimate goal. To achieve the abs you want, you have to be able to clearly see the goal in your mind's eye. The vision could be based on a picture from a magazine, the way you looked when you were on the college wrestling team, someone you saw at the beach, or any combination of these things. What's important is that you create a specific image of how you want your abs to look.

The creation of this mental picture is a tool called visualization. Consciously creating a positive image can actually help you achieve your goal of a strong midsection.

Most of the world's greatest athletes use visualization. In fact, athletes were visualizing long before anyone gave it a name. Jack Nicklaus mentally previews each golf shot before he takes his backswing. Divers, dancers, and gymnasts all know the value of mentally practicing before performing.

Most successful athletes use some form of visualization to help them perform better, as do most successful business people. In fact, successful people in all walks of life usually use some form of visualization in achieving their goals. We all do it when we dream of the future: a new car, a big house in the country, a hole in one. Visualization is a skill that works for everyone, the elite athlete and the struggling novice.

One study involving basketball free throws illustrates the effectiveness of visualization. A group of study subjects who spent 20 minutes a day for 20 days visualizing themselves successfully making free throws showed a 23 percent increase over the number of free throws they were able to make at the start of the study. This was nearly as big of an improvement as that of a group who actually practiced shooting a real ball for 20 minutes a day, 20 days in a row—that group improved by 24 percent. By contrast, a third group who engaged in neither physical practice nor visualization showed no improvement at all.

The reason that visualization works is simple. Your brain can't tell the difference between a real event and an imagined one, so by using your imagination, you can create positive experiences that improve your self-image and your skills.

## HAVING A VISION

Here are some tips to help you make your visualization of your new body as effective as possible.

**Be true to yourself.** It is important to keep an element of truth and realism in your picture. Create an image of your body that fits your genetic type and potential. It must be a vision that you can believe with every cell of your body, not one that will be impossible to achieve.

**Pay attention to detail.** Make the snapshot of your ideal abs as specific as possible. The more vivid the visualization, the more effective it will be. See every line of defin-ition in your abs. See both the separation of your muscles and the way your muscles attach to each other. It is essential to use many layers of sensory detail. See the color of your skin and the way your muscles move under it. Imagine the way your muscles feel when you touch them and move them. Taste the relief of cold water or a sports drink when you do a great workout. Hear your friends telling you that you're looking pretty good and your lover complimenting your body. And see the beautiful stranger turning to watch you as you walk by.

**Take a vote of confidence.** Your visualization should also include your improved emotional well-being. Feel your increased self-confidence and your sustained motivation.

**Be a dedicated viewer.** You must visualize every day, not just on occasion. Your mind is just like a muscle. You have to work it consistently if you expect it to develop. But you are not locked into one image forever. Your picture can change, evolve, and refine itself as you get closer to your goal.

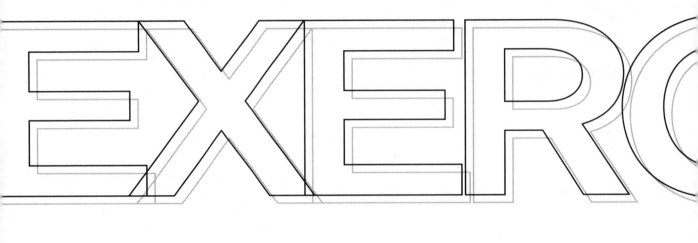

# PART TWO

# CISE
# ESSENTIALS

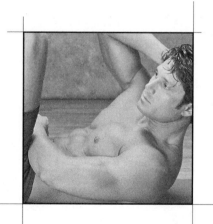

# ESSENTIAL
# PHYSIOLOGY

You don't have to be an expert in anatomy and physiology to trim your waist and build and strengthen the muscles in your midsection. But if you're going to do the work it takes to make changes in your body, you should at least be able to visualize the objects of your effort. This chapter will explain and illustrate the primary muscles you'll be training—and you won't need a Ph.D. to understand it.

## YOUR MUSCLES

**Rectus abdominis.** This muscle pulls your torso toward your hips, as in a crunch, and your hips toward your torso, as in a reverse crunch.

When people talk about abs, they're usually talking about this large strip of muscle that runs from your pubic bone to your sternum. On most people, a perfectly developed rectus abdominis has six segments of muscle above the belly button (the "six-pack," or upper abs) and a flat sheath below (the lower abs). The terms *upper abs* and *lower abs* are therefore slightly inaccurate since the rectus abdominis is really one muscle. But the sensation in the muscle when you do crunches (which work its upper, segmented portion) is different from the feeling you have when you do reverse crunches (which engage the lower, flat section). So it's easiest to talk about the rectus in terms of where you feel the effort when you exercise.

Thanks to individual genetics, you could have a four-pack or even an eight-pack above your navel instead of a six-pack. Or you could have six segments aligned asymmetrically: The panels on one side could be slightly higher than the ones on the other side. If you get to the point where you discover that your rectus abdominis has an odd structure or symmetry, you should congratulate yourself—you have to be in damned good shape to see the muscle clearly enough to notice.

**External and internal obliques.** These muscles twist your body at the waist, as in crossovers, and straighten your torso when it's bent to the side, as in side bends.

The obliques run from the front halves of your hips and the crest of your pubic bone up to your ribs (just below your chest). They also attach to the rectus abdominis and the serratus (the muscles that cover the sides of your ribs).

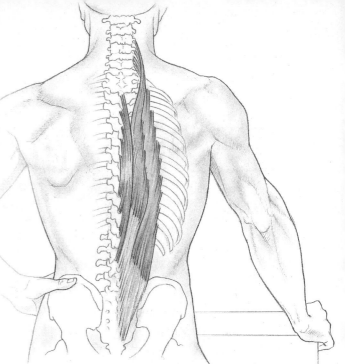

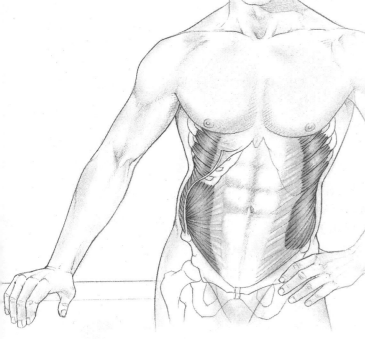

Aesthetically, the obliques frame and highlight the rectus abdominis, shaping your torso as it rises from your hips to your chest. Functionally, the obliques are crucial in sports that involve twisting at the waist—baseball, golf, hockey, and racket sports, for example.

The internal oblique lies underneath the external oblique and runs diagonally in the opposite direction. Although it aids in twisting, it's also a postural muscle that contracts to keep your torso upright.

**Spinal erectors.** These muscles in your lower back straighten your body when it's bent forward at the waist, assist in twisting your body at the waist, and protect your spine.

Nobody starts an exercise program with hopes of getting great-looking spinal erectors, but these muscles are crucial to your day-to-day feeling of health and vitality. Sitting all day weakens the muscles and stretches out the connective tissues in your lower back, making you feel drained when you get home. Strengthening your lower back and abdominals in tandem will improve your posture, make sitting more comfortable, and leave you with energy at the end of the day.

## BODY MECHANICS

Exercise success is a matter of feeling. If you don't know what you're supposed to feel, you'll just go through the motions and never fully activate the muscles you're trying to work. Here are the principles of body alignment and exercise technique for your ab muscles and lower back that will help ensure that you get the best results from your exercises.

### Upper Abs

**What you do:** You make two basic movements when you emphasize your upper abs in exercises like crunches: You bring your shoulder blades forward (1) and you move your rib cage toward your hips (2).

**What you should feel:** Upper-ab exercises should cause a squeezing sensation in the muscles just below your rib cage.

**Practice this:** While sitting, try to pull your rib cage down toward your belly button without consciously leaning forward.

### Lower Abs

**What you do:** Your lower abs are activated in movements like a hip up. You rotate your hips upward, toward your rib cage (3).

**What you should feel:** Lower-ab work should result in a squeezing sensation below your belly button.

**Practice this:** Pretend, for a second, that you're a Chippendales dancer. (Make sure that you're alone in the room, with the blinds closed.) Thrust your pelvis forward and upward as if you were trying to drive a crowd of ovulating women into a hormonal frenzy. Then take your thighs and buttocks out of the action, and try to move only your pelvis. Those are your lower abs in action. Okay, open the blinds, sit down, and pretend nothing happened, even though your life will never be the same.

### Obliques

**What you do:** These muscles are exercised in movements like a crossover. You move one shoulder blade forward and turn it toward the opposite hip (see photo 4 on page 34).

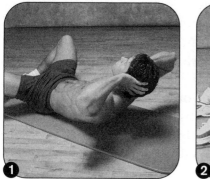
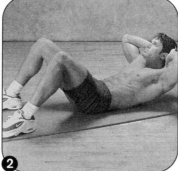
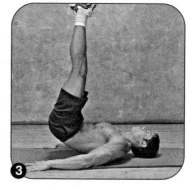

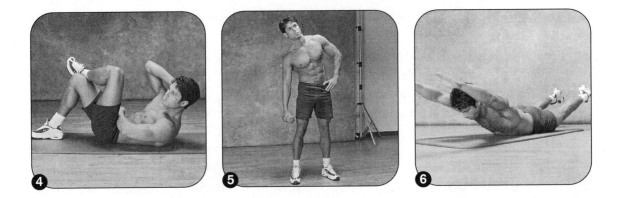

You also work your obliques when you do side bends, which move your rib cage directly toward the side of your hip (5).

**What you should feel:** If you're moving from your right side to your left, you should feel a squeeze all along the right side of your abdomen, but it should be most intense a couple of inches to the right of your belly button. When moving from left to right, the sensation should be on your left.

**Practice this:** Sitting or standing, hold your right hand to your right ear. Crunch your rib cage down toward your hip as you twist slightly to your left. Keep trying it from different angles, with slight variations on the twisting motion, until you feel that squeeze just to the right of your umbilicus. Then switch sides and practice until you feel the squeeze just to the left of your belly button.

Remember, if you hold a weight in your right hand when you do an oblique exercise, you work the oblique muscles on the left side of your torso. Lowering the weight stretches the muscles on your left side, not those on your right side. It's when you straighten your body that you should feel the squeezing sensation in your left obliques.

## Spinal Erectors

**What you do:** Exercises like superman work your spinal erectors. These muscles are activated when you straighten your lower back when it's curled forward (6).

**What you should feel:** Lower-back exercises should cause a tightening in the muscles on either side of your spine below your rib cage.

**Practice this:** Sit in a chair—preferably in front of your computer keyboard—and slouch. In other words, sit as you usually do. Then, pretend that your boss/paramour/drill sergeant has just walked into the room, and sit at attention, bolt upright. Notice how your lower-back muscles tighten to get you out of your slouch. Other muscles are involved—your trapezius in your upper back pulls your shoulders back, for example—but tightening your spinal erectors has the biggest effect in taking you from slumped to straight.

# ESSENTIAL FLEXIBILITY
## STRETCHES

Flexibility is the missing element in many guys' fitness programs. Guys who lift diligently, sweat out liters during their aerobic work, and choose mustard instead of mayonnaise on their turkey sandwiches will often skip stretching. They figure that stretching just takes up time that could be better devoted to "real" exercise.

Don't be one of those guys. A preworkout stretching routine will improve your performance in any activity requiring strength, balance, and power—from crunches to weight lifting to sex. More important, a flexible body is a more comfortable body to walk around in all day. Regular stretching will ease tension in your muscles and joints and improve your posture (all the better to show off those abs).

## AB-SPECIFIC FLEXIBILITY

The stretches on the following pages focus on your neck, shoulders, and back. They'll help you improve your range of motion in abdominal work. A bigger range of motion means better gains. In other words, flexibility equals muscle.

Do these five routines after a 5-minute warmup and before your ab exercises. Hold each stretch for 10 seconds. After completing each exercise, move on to the next without resting. The entire stretching workout should take you less than 5 minutes.

# Neck-Stretch Series

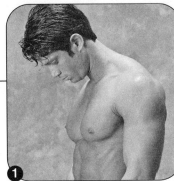 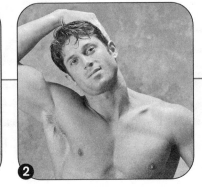 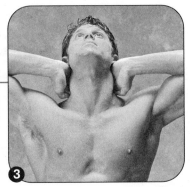

### READY, SET, GO:

**1.** Drop your head forward, chin to chest.

**2.** Place your right hand on the left side of your head, just above your ear. Lower your right ear toward your right shoulder, using your hand to gently assist. Repeat to the left.

**3.** Place your hands behind your neck with your fingertips touching, and gently tilt your head back, using your hands for support. Don't crunch your neck back and compress your vertebrae.

# Shoulder-Stretch Series

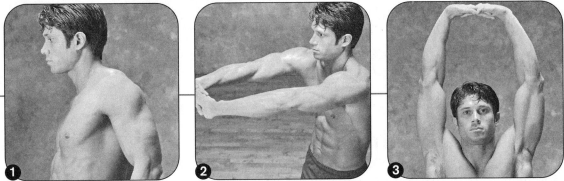

### READY, SET, GO:

**1.** Raise your shoulders toward your ears and slowly roll them backward. Do this five times. Then, slowly roll your shoulders forward five times.

**2.** Extend your arms in front of your body, interlocking your fingers and turning your palms away from you. Round your upper back as you press your palms outward.

**3.** Keeping your fingers interlocked, straighten your back and extend your arms over your head, pressing your palms up toward the ceiling.

# Side Bend

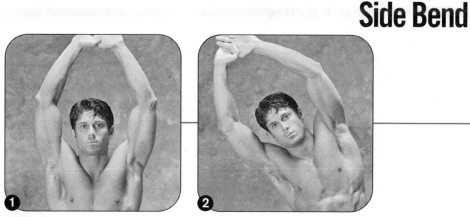

**READY, SET, GO:**

**1.** Stand with your feet together, your arms fully extended over your head, and your thumbs interlocked.

**2.** Lengthen and bend over your right side. Repeat to your left side.

# Torso-and-Hamstring Series

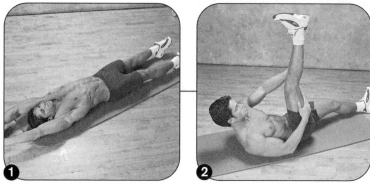

**READY, SET, GO:**

**1.** Lie on your back with your arms extended over your head and your legs fully extended on the floor. Stretch your entire body, from your fingertips to your toes, trying to lengthen your body in both directions.

**2.** Lift your right leg and grab it with both hands. Gently pull it toward your head. You may find it helpful to raise your head, bringing your chin to your chest. Repeat with your left leg.

# Lower-Back Series

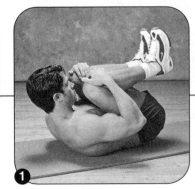 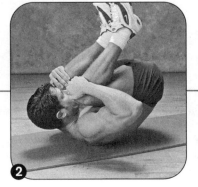 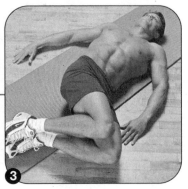

**READY, SET, GO:**

**1.** Lie on your back and bring both knees to your chest. Grab both knees and gently pull them toward your shoulders. At the same time, tuck your head and bring your chin to your chest.

**2.** Gently and slowly, roll back and forth five times. *Caution:* You need a mat or well-padded and carpeted floor to do this safely.

**3.** Set your feet on the floor and let both legs fall to your left side. Repeat to your right side.

# CHAPTER SEVEN

# ESSENTIAL
# TECHNIQUES

The last thing I want to do is blitz you with a hundred technical details to keep in mind while you're trying to do a few simple abdominal exercises. But you do need some basic knowledge to exercise injury-free and achieve the best results in the least amount of time. So let's start with a few simple guidelines to make your workouts more productive and fun. Here are eight rules for abdominal exercise.

## #1
## ALWAYS WARM UP

You're not exactly a rebel if you don't warm up before you train your abs. Most guys probably don't. Some guys even use ab exercises as a warmup for the rest of their workout. Other well-intentioned guys find that it's a challenge to just get down on the floor and crank out a set of crunches before bed—let alone do a warmup first. There's nothing wrong with that. Small victories add up. Doing a little exercise is always better than doing nothing. But no matter what kind of exercise you're doing, you won't get the best possible results unless your body is prepared. Here's what a warmup can add to your workout.

■ It turns up the heat, literally increasing the temperature in your muscles and connective tissues. Warm muscles are more pliable, and pliable muscles can accomplish more.

- It fills your muscles with blood. This gives the muscles more fuel and, thus, more power. The muscles can now work harder and faster.
- Finally, a good warmup can help clear your mind of distractions and focus it on the task you're about to perform—in this case, abdominal exercises.

A warmup doesn't have to be the formal 5-minutes-on-a-treadmill routine that you see everyone in the gym doing. (And that's not even an option if you exercise at home and don't have a few thousand bucks to lay out for a decent treadmill.) Here are a few other options.

**Play.** Play ball with your kids, walk or run around with the dog, or just put on some rock 'n' roll and shake your money-maker.

**Get something done around the house.** Your wife or roommate will love this option. Take out the trash, do the laundry, pick up the kids' toys. Just make sure it's something that keeps you moving from room to room.

**If all else fails, just exercise.** Jump rope, jog in place, do some jumping jacks. These exercises are actually kind of fun to do as an adult, when you're many years removed from junior-high P.E. class.

## #2
## USE A FULL RANGE OF MOTION

To get the full benefit of an exercise, you need to go through a full range of motion. On crunches, this means raising your shoulder blades off the floor on each repetition and curling your rib cage toward your hips. Moving your head up and down in a nodding motion is not a full range of motion—in fact, it's not even an exercise.

## #3
## CONTROL THE SPEED OF EACH REPETITION

The point of exercise is to work against gravity, not let gravity control your movement. So when you do abdominal exercises, you need to control your speed as you raise your body (this is called the positive, or concentric, part of the exercise) and while you lower it (called the negative, or eccentric, portion).

You get a muscle-building effect during both the positive and negative parts of the exercise. Skipping the negative portion by letting your body flop back to the floor is cheating yourself out of half of the exercise's benefits.

## #4
## BREATHE WHILE EXERCISING

Sure, it sounds obvious. But ask any trainer how many beginners instinctively breathe while doing abdominal exercises, and the answer will probably hover around zero. Almost all of us, when we're starting out, hold our breath the first few times we do crunches.

Here's the ideal way to breathe during exercise. Near the end of the positive phase of each repetition, exhale through your mouth. In a crunch, you exhale as you raise your shoulder blades off the floor. Inhale through your nose during the negative phase. In a crunch, you inhale as you lower your torso back toward the floor.

That said, it's also important to note that in abdominal exercises, the range of motion is pretty small—sometimes just a couple of inches. So a strict breathing pattern may feel unnatural. You may find yourself exhaling on the negative phase and inhaling on the positive. You know what? It won't hurt your progress at all. Just don't hold your breath.

### #5
## ALWAYS CHOOSE QUALITY OVER QUANTITY

Every gym has a few guys who do thousands of sloppy-ass crunches and think they're accomplishing something. But the best predictor of success in abdominal exercise is not how much you do but how

## A FEW WORDS ABOUT AB ROLLERS

Ask any trainer about ab rollers, and he'll probably give you one of the following two responses:

■ They're a crutch. People are much better off just getting down on the floor and learning to do the standard exercises.

■ They're not great, but at least they get people to start exercising.

Most people who have ab rollers probably bought them because they thought that the devices would magically make abdominal exercises easier. But ab rollers present a whole new set of challenges. If you already own one,

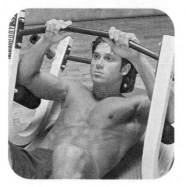

here's how to get the most out of it.

**1.** Make sure the neck pad does not drive your head toward your chest, putting strain on your neck. Keep a fist's distance between your chin and chest, and let your neck relax into the pad.

**2.** Don't push the roller down with your elbows. That turns a good abdominal movement into a mediocre chest-and-back exercise.

**3.** Don't push the roller down with your hands or grip it tightly. Doing so makes your brain focus on your hands and forearms rather than on your abdominals. If you're not thinking about your abdominals, you're not working them effectively.

**4.** Don't let the unit creep forward. If it does, you're working muscles other than your abdominals.

**5.** Control the roller; don't let it control you. In other words, don't let momentum take over. You still need to control both the upward and downward phases of the movement.

well you do it. Two keys to doing ab exercises well are to make sure you feel a contraction—a squeezing sensation—in your midsection on every repetition and to maintain constant tension in your ab muscles throughout the positive and negative portions of each repetition.

So now another question arises: What happens if you stop feeling that squeeze on your repetitions, if you can't keep tension on your muscles?

Quit. Stop the set.

But what if you're not finished with the set?

When you can't maintain the tension on your muscles anymore, the set is finished. It doesn't matter how many repetitions you've done or how many more you think you have to do. When the thrill is gone, the set is over.

Let's take a closer look at what happens when you near the end of a set. Say you're going for 15 repetitions but find that on the 10th rep, you start to struggle. On rep 11, your ab muscles burn as you barely get your shoulder blades off the floor. On rep 12, you rest on the floor for a moment. Then, in an explosive, jerky motion, you pull your head forward, trying to get your shoulder blades up.

Okay, you're done. The set is over. You've had a breakdown in technique—you tried but couldn't do any more repetitions with good form. Since there's no point in continuing with bad form, you should congratulate yourself for pushing your body as hard as it could go, and move on to the next exercise in your workout.

## #6
## EXERCISE THROUGH GOOD PAIN AND STOP WHEN YOU FEEL BAD PAIN

It's normal to feel some discomfort at the end of a set. Your ab muscles will burn, your body will probably shake, your breathing will get ragged. That's good pain. You don't have to push yourself that hard on every set to get results—in fact, you shouldn't. But you have to know where your limits are in order to signal to your body that you want to improve beyond them.

Good pain is your sign that you're reaching those limits. And believe it or not, the more you exercise, the more you'll rely on good pain to let you know how you're doing. You may not ever find it pleasurable, but you'll know that it's good that you feel it.

Bad pain is a warning sign. It means you've injured yourself. Some bad pains include shooting pains, sharp pains, spasms, and pain that moves beyond the muscles you're exercising.

If you feel any of these, stop your set and try to figure out what happened. Try to move and stretch the area where the pain originated. When you're doing ab exercises, that area will most likely be your neck or lower back. If you're still sore after stretching, that's it. Your workout is over. Continuing just guarantees that you'll hurt yourself worse and need to put in time on the couch or, worse, the doctor's table. And that puts you further from your goal of improving your fitness level.

# 7

# ISOLATE THE PART OF YOUR ABDOMINALS THAT YOU'RE TRAINING

The exercises in this book are intended to isolate different parts of your midsection—upper abs, lower abs, and obliques. The key is to make sure that in each repetition you feel the contraction in the area that you're targeting. Sometimes you'll feel an exercise working in two places at once. For example, you'll feel a crossover first in your upper abs and then in your obliques.

Sloppy technique is your enemy. If you don't do the exercise right, you won't feel the isolated contraction. The following sloppy practices are on the most-wanted list.

## Upper-Ab Movements

**Problem:** You just move your neck up and down instead of moving your shoulder blades off the floor.

**Solution:** Initiate the movement with your ab muscles, pulling your rib cage toward your hips and allowing your head to follow the action rather than lead it.

**Problem:** You use your arms to pull your head and torso forward, hoping your shoulder blades will follow.

**Solution:** Support your head with just your fingertips, and make your abs lift your shoulder blades off the floor.

## Lower-Ab Movements

**Problem:** You move your knees toward your chest but don't get your hips to curl off the floor toward your rib cage.

**Solution:** Start the movement in your lower abdominal muscles, not in your legs. You want your ab muscles to force your hips and legs to move.

Sometimes it's hard to figure out if your hips are actually curling off the floor. An easy trick is to place your fingertips at the edges of your hips so you can feel your hips curl up.

**Problem:** You use a rocking motion or push off with your hands to get your hips off the floor.

**Solution:** Keep your arms and hands relaxed, not flexed and ready for action.

## Oblique Movements

**Problem:** Instead of lifting your shoulder blade off the floor on a crossover, you just flap your arm toward your opposite knee.

**Solution:** Perform two actions: First, raise your shoulder blade off the floor, then twist your shoulder across. That's up, then across.

**Problem:** You shift your weight in one direction to gain momentum in the opposite direction. For example, on a crossover, you shift your body weight to the right so you can bounce or rebound to the left. This is instinctive—if you were going to jump, you'd first lower your body, then quickly spring upward. Or if you were going to try to push a stalled car, you'd lean back before pushing against the car's bumper.

**Solution:** This gets back to the point about controlling the exercise at both phases, going up and coming down. If you have your body under control at all times, you won't use bouncing and jerking movements to perform the exercise.

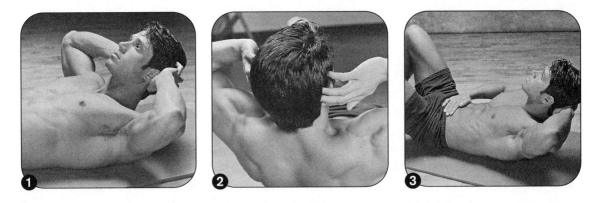

## #8
## WATCH YOUR NECK

Neck discomfort is a potential problem during abdominal exercises. But the problem isn't really your neck; that's just where you feel the problem. The offender is that big ol' head of yours, weighing in at between 8 and 10 pounds. Lifting that thing up and down is a tough chore for your neck. However, most guys find that their necks get stronger the longer they do abdominal exercises.

Here are some neck-saving tips.

**When doing ab work, always maintain a space about the size of your fist between your chin and chest (1).** Keep the integrity of this space throughout the entire movement—don't pull your head forward. Pay special attention to this placement as you start to get tired.

## EXERCISE TO HOLD YOUR HEAD HIGH

You can keep your ab workout from becoming a real pain in the neck with this simple neck-strengthening exercise.

Lie on a weight bench or your bed so your head and neck hang off the edge with no support. Use your neck muscles to hold your head up so it's in a straight line with your spine, as if you were standing.

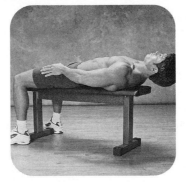

Start off by holding this position for 5 seconds, then increase the duration by 5 seconds each time you exercise until you can hold it for a full minute. If you can't increase it by 5 seconds each time, that's fine; go at your own pace.

Do this exercise twice a week. If you do it on one of your ab-workout days, do it after your ab exercises or at a different time entirely.

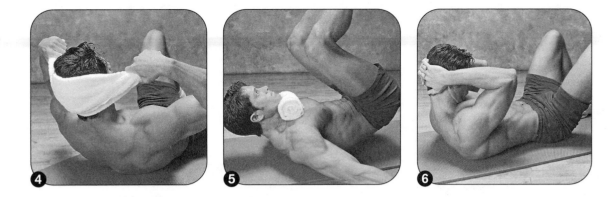

**Support your head with your hands or a towel.** If you use your hands, place your fingertips behind your ears (2). This signals your neck muscles to release some tension.

Or cup your head with one hand, and put your free hand on the part of your midsection that you're targeting (3). Feel the muscles contract and release. This technique serves two purposes: It lets you support your head, taking tension off your neck, and also allows you to feel your abdominal muscles at work.

For best results when using a towel to do upper-ab exercises, spread the towel out, creating a wide web to support your head (4). This works only if you keep your hands in a fixed position relative to your head. If you use your hands to pull the towel—and your head—forward, you're straining your neck, not supporting it.

When doing reverse crunches, you can put a rolled-up towel beneath your chin (5). This helps keep the proper distance between your chin and chest.

**Don't interlace your fingers behind your head.** As with pulling on the towel behind your head, interlacing your fingers and pulling your head forward only serves to drive your chin toward your chest, straining your neck (6).

## EXERCISING WITH INTEGRITY
Proper technique boils down to this: You're responsible for the integrity of the movement. It doesn't matter if you're doing abdominal exercises on the floor next to your bed, on an expensive health-club machine, or on a cheap infomercial gizmo. It's still all you. The more you're in control of the exercise, the more you get out of it.

Using machines seems easier than doing floor exercises, but in reality it's not. You still have to do the work, no matter how much metal you've strapped yourself to.

That's why *Essential Abs* starts you off with no-frills floor exercises. They'll teach you control and discipline and help you connect your mind to the muscles you're working. That's the key to success, to getting the results you want from the effort you expend.

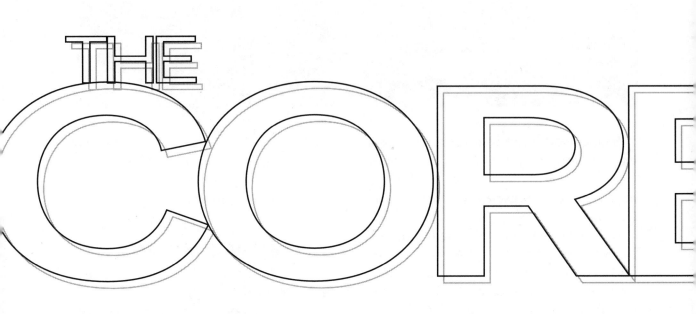

THE CORE

# PART THREE

# PROGRAM

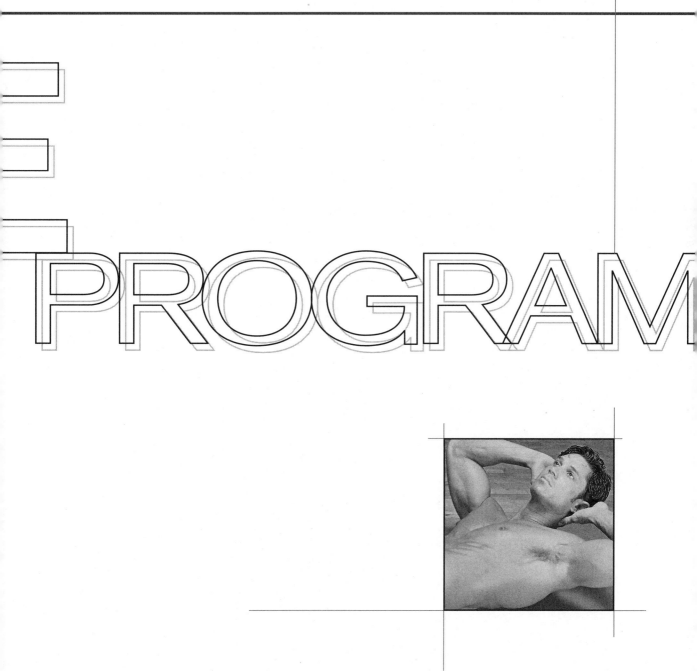

# CHAPTER EIGHT

# ESSENTIAL KNOWLEDGE

The *Essential Abs* Core Program will take you from doing no exercise to doing about 3 hours a week. By the end of the 6-week Core Program, you'll be doing a full workout of abdominal and aerobic exercises—enough of each to develop the muscles in your midsection and lower back and improve your cardiovascular health.

The Core Program is a simple and effective series of routines designed to help you create a positive exercise habit. The 6-week system is just a template. You may need longer than the suggested 2 weeks before you're able to complete the recommended number of repetitions for a particular exercise at a given level, and you may have to rest between exercises. It might take some guys 9 weeks to complete the Core Program, while others might take 3 months. But your strength and endurance will gradually increase as you progress through the program.

Although the program is progressive, you don't have to conquer all three levels to gain substantial benefits. Your lifestyle and fitness goals might be satisfied by completing just Level One. Or you might stay at Level Two for a few months before tackling Level Three. Everyone is different. Adjust the template to fit your lifestyle and needs.

Safety is the most important consideration when learning new exercises. If you have any special health issues or concerns, make sure you consult a physician before you start the program.

Use this chart to help you monitor your progress through the Core Program. In the "Workout" columns, the numbers on the left sides of the slashes are the rec-

| | WEEK 1 | | | |
|---|---|---|---|---|
| **LEVEL-ONE EXERCISES** | **WORKOUT 1** | **WORKOUT 2** | **WORKOUT 3** | **WORKOUT 4** |
| Reverse crunch | 12/ | 13/ | 14/ | — |
| Crossover | 12/ | 13/ | 14/ | — |
| Crunch: feet flat | 12/ | 13/ | 14/ | — |
| Opposite arm and leg raise | 12/ | 13/ | 14/ | — |
| **LEVEL-TWO EXERCISES** | **WORKOUT 1** | **WORKOUT 2** | **WORKOUT 3** | **WORKOUT 4** |
| Hip up | 12/ | 13/ | 14/ | — |
| Reverse crunch | 12/ | 13/ | 14/ | — |
| Crossover | 12/ | 13/ | 14/ | — |
| Oblique crunch | 12/ | 13/ | 14/ | — |
| Crunch: legs up | 12/ | 13/ | 14/ | — |
| Crunch: feet flat | 12/ | 13/ | 14/ | — |
| Superman | 12/ | 13/ | 14/ | — |
| **LEVEL-THREE EXERCISES** | **WORKOUT 1** | **WORKOUT 2** | **WORKOUT 3** | **WORKOUT 4** |
| Corkscrew | 12/ | 12/ | 13/ | 13/ |
| Hip up | 12/ | 12/ | 13/ | 13/ |
| Reverse crunch | 12/ | 12/ | 13/ | 13/ |
| Crossover | 12/ | 12/ | 13/ | 13/ |
| Oblique crunch | 12/ | 12/ | 13/ | 13/ |
| Catch | 12/ | 12/ | 13/ | 13/ |
| Toe touch | 12/ | 12/ | 13/ | 13/ |
| Crunch: legs up | 12/ | 12/ | 13/ | 13/ |
| Crunch: frog legs | 12/ | 12/ | 13/ | 13/ |
| Isometric back extension | 4 (4 sec holds)/ | 5 (4 sec holds)/ | 6 (4 sec holds)/ | 6 (4 sec holds)/ |

ommended number of repetitions. Track how many reps
you actually finish by
recording those numbers to
the right sides of the
slashes.

| WORKOUT 1 | WORKOUT 2 | WORKOUT 3 | WORKOUT 4 |
|---|---|---|---|
| 16/ | 17/ | 18/ | — |
| 16/ | 17/ | 18/ | — |
| 16/ | 17/ | 18/ | — |
| 16/ | 17/ | 18/ | — |

| WORKOUT 1 | WORKOUT 2 | WORKOUT 3 | WORKOUT 4 |
|---|---|---|---|
| 16/ | 17/ | 18/ | — |
| 16/ | 17/ | 18/ | — |
| 16/ | 17/ | 18/ | — |
| 16/ | 17/ | 18/ | — |
| 16/ | 17/ | 18/ | — |
| 16/ | 17/ | 18/ | — |
| 16/ | 17/ | 18/ | — |

| WORKOUT 1 | WORKOUT 2 | WORKOUT 3 | WORKOUT 4 |
|---|---|---|---|
| 14/ | 14/ | 15/ | 15/ |
| 14/ | 14/ | 15/ | 15/ |
| 14/ | 14/ | 15/ | 15/ |
| 14/ | 14/ | 15/ | 15/ |
| 14/ | 14/ | 15/ | 15/ |
| 14/ | 14/ | 15/ | 15/ |
| 14/ | 14/ | 15/ | 15/ |
| 14/ | 14/ | 15/ | 15/ |
| 14/ | 14/ | 15/ | 15/ |
| 5 (5 sec holds)/ | 6 (5 sec holds)/ | 7 (5 sec holds)/ | 7 (5 sec holds)/ |

It is especially important not to push yourself too hard. Your main focus should be on mastering proper technique. Focus on technique until you can do the movement correctly without thinking. When learning a new movement, practice it while you are fresh. In other words, don't try to learn it late at night or at the end of a workout, when you are exhausted. This can lead to unnecessary frustration and excessive soreness.

To help you refine your technique, each abs exercise in the program is accompanied by performance tips that are specific to that particular exercise. Here are some general reminders that you can apply to every exercise.

## Performance Tips

- Keep constant tension on your abs.
- Keep each motion slow and controlled, with no bouncing or jerking, for both the positive and negative phases of the movement.
- Pause for a total contraction at the top of the movement.
- Don't rest between repetitions.
- Focus on feeling your abs doing the work, putting your mind in your muscle. Don't just go through the motions.
- Let your head relax into your hands or a towel, taking stress off your neck.
- Remember to keep breathing; don't hold your breath.

## BEYOND THE EXERCISES

At each level, the ab routine is supplemented by a troubleshooting section that addresses common problems and answers frequently asked questions.

On top of that, each of the three levels of the Core Program offers tips on aerobic exercise and eating better. By the end of the program, you'll be not only exercising your abs but also doing cardiovascular work and modifying your diet so that you get visible results much faster.

By the end of the Core Program, you will have learned the ab essentials that you need to have the fit midsection that you want, and you will be well on your way to getting it. So why waste any more time? Let's get started.

# CHAPTER NINE

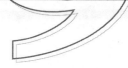

# ESSENTIAL
## FIRST STEP
### LEVEL ONE

In Level One of the Core Program, you really have just one goal: getting to Level Two. Here's what you have to do to achieve that goal.

■ Do three abdominal exercises and one lower-back exercise three times a week.
■ Add some easy cardiovascular exercise in the second week.
■ Think about how you're eating now, and try to incorporate some of our simple suggestions for eating smarter.

## THE LEVEL-ONE ROUTINE
■ Do this routine three times a week.
■ Do one set of each exercise.
■ Do 12 repetitions of each exercise in your first workout, 13 in your second, and 14 in your third. The next week, start with 16 reps of each and work up to 18.
■ Between exercises, try to rest for no longer than 5 seconds. If you have to rest more, that's fine; but try to decrease your rest time with each workout.

**BENEFITS**
OF LEVEL ONE

More strength in your abdominal muscles

Less discomfort in your lower back, if you currently have problems in that area

Better posture

# Reverse Crunch

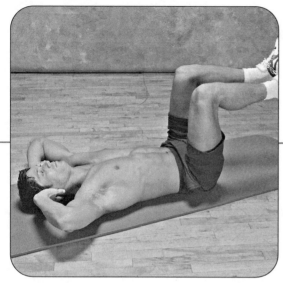
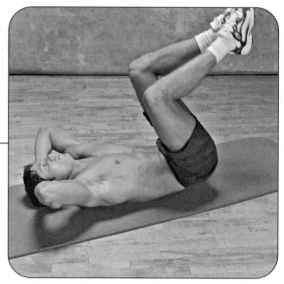

**READY, SET:**

Lie on your back with your head and neck relaxed and your hands behind your ears. You want your lower body to form two right angles: Your thighs should be perpendicular to your upper body, with your lower legs parallel to the floor.

**GO:**

Use your lower abs to raise your hips off the floor and toward your rib cage.

Then, in a controlled motion, slowly lower your hips back to the starting position. As they lightly touch the floor, repeat.

## PERFORMANCE TIPS

- Make sure your lower abs do the work. If you rock up and down, you're using momentum to aid you in the exercise, taking work away from your lower abs.

- Don't rest your hips on the floor at the bottom of the movement or let your lower legs drop down.

- Keep constant tension on your abs.

- Use your hands for balance. Don't use them to push off.

- Keep your head and neck relaxed.

# Crossover

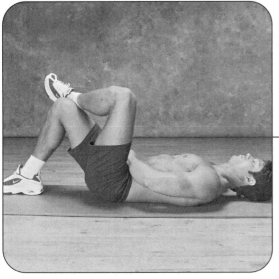

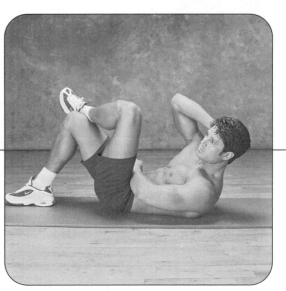

## READY, SET:

Lie on your back with your knees up and your feet on the floor. Cross your left leg over your right leg. Your left ankle should rest just below your right knee, making a triangle between your legs. Put your right hand behind your head, with your elbow extended to the side. Rest your head and elbow on the floor. Place your left hand on your right obliques or at your left side.

## GO:

Use your right obliques to raise your right shoulder and cross it toward your left knee.

Then, in a controlled motion, slowly lower your shoulder back to the starting position. As soon as your shoulder blade lightly touches the floor, repeat.

When you finish all of your repetitions on your right side, switch positions to work your left side: Put your right ankle below your left knee, put your left hand behind your head, and raise your left shoulder toward your right knee. Do the same number of reps on your left side.

## PERFORMANCE TIPS

- Make sure that your entire torso twists up and toward your knee. Don't just move your elbow or shoulder. Don't move your knee toward your shoulder.

- Feel the squeeze in your oblique muscles on the side that you're working. You'll probably also feel it in your upper abs on that side, which is fine.

- Move up and down slowly; don't use momentum to finish your repetitions.

# Crunch: Feet Flat

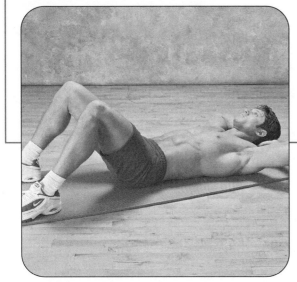 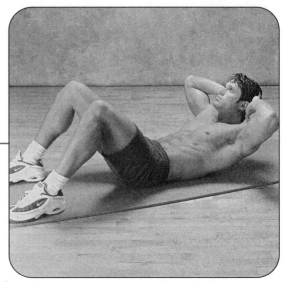

**READY, SET:**

Lie on your back with your knees bent, your feet flat on the floor, your head and neck relaxed, and your hands behind your ears.

**GO:**

Use your upper abs to raise your rib cage toward your pelvis and lift your shoulder blades off the floor. Hold for a second.

Then, in a controlled motion, slowly lower your shoulders back to the starting position. As soon as your shoulder blades lightly touch the floor, repeat.

## PERFORMANCE TIPS

■ Make sure your shoulder blades come off the floor each time. Don't just move your head and neck.

■ Move up and down slowly; don't use momentum to finish your repetitions.

■ Keep constant tension on your abs throughout the movement—don't rest at the bottom of the movement.

■ Pause at the top of the movement, after you've exhaled, and feel the squeeze go deeper into your abdominals.

# Opposite Arm and Leg Raise

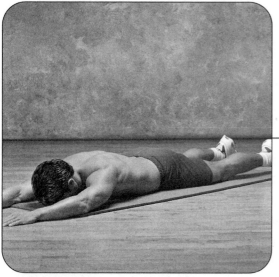 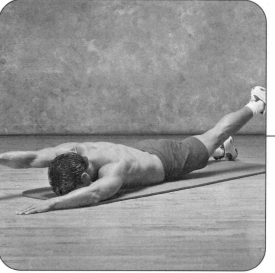

## READY, SET:

Lie facedown on the floor with your arms and legs extended. Your palms should face the floor.

## GO:

Simultaneously raise your right arm and left leg to a comfortable height. Hold for 2 seconds.

Then, in a contolled motion, slowly return to the starting position. As soon as your arm and leg lightly touch the floor, repeat with your left arm and right leg. Alternate until you've done all the recommended repetitions on each side.

## PERFORMANCE TIPS

■ As you raise your arm and leg, also try to extend them—that is, make them reach out farther.

■ You'll also feel this exercise in your gluteals and hamstrings as you raise your legs.

■ If it feels too easy to simply raise one arm and leg, try keeping your nonworking arm and leg off the floor throughout the exercise. So while you raise your right arm and left leg, keep your left arm and right leg off the floor slightly. Then, as you lift the latter limbs, stop short of touching your right arm and left leg to the floor. That will keep more tension on your lower back throughout the set.

■ When I train my abs, my neck hurts more than my stomach.

Neck pain is common when you're just starting out. Ab work puts some stress on your neck muscles, which may be very weak. Just like any other muscle, your neck will fatigue and become sore. It's natural—soreness, if it's not preceded or accompanied by sharp pain, is simply a sign that you've worked a muscle in a way in which it's not used to being worked. The muscles in your neck will quickly get stronger, and you'll stop getting sore.

■ I can't do the recommended number of repetitions. It's very discouraging.

The recommended repetitions are just initial goals. For some exercisers, they'll be a little too challenging, and for others, they'll be a little too easy (see below). Stay with it, and your numbers will rise. If you have to, stick with Level One beyond the first 2 weeks. Keep at it until you can do the suggested number of repetitions with good form.

■ These exercises don't feel very challenging. I can easily do 20 repetitions of each exercise.

You have two choices: One, jump ahead to Level Two or even Level Three since you are obviously in pretty good shape and have a body that's ready for more strenuous exercise. Or, two, challenge yourself to do the exercises as slowly as possible. On each repetition, hold the middle position—the point at which your muscles are fully contracted—for 2 or 3 seconds. Then take another 2 or 3 seconds to lower yourself. Even very experienced exercisers will have trouble completing 12 repetitions using those parameters.

■ It doesn't feel like anything is happening in my lower abs.

When you're trying to work the lower section of the rectus abdominis, it's easy to recruit other muscles to help. The hip flexors, small muscles on the sides of your pelvis, are notorious for offering unwanted assistance in lower-abdominal exercises. The key is to isolate your lower abs. Do these exercises first in your workouts (they're listed first throughout the Core Program). Start lower-ab movements by lifting your pelvis up off the floor an inch or two, then curling it toward your rib cage.

## GET UP AND MOVE

Firm abdominal muscles are nice to have, but the number one muscle in your body is your heart. Your heart's condition is a strong indicator of how long and how well you'll live. A stronger and more efficient heart will improve your performance and make work and recreation more enjoyable.

How do you make your heart stronger? You move. Activities like walking, jogging, biking, and swimming are all classic examples of aerobic exercise because they all increase your heart rate and respiration. This type of exercise also improves your circulation, lowers your blood pressure and resting heart rate, and helps you lose weight.

## HOW LONG, HOW HARD?

If you're really out of shape, any steady movement will improve your cardiovascular fitness. (You'll notice that we use the words *cardiovascular* and *aerobic* interchangeably in this book. They both mean exercise in which your body moves at a pace that requires your heart to pump faster than it would if you were resting.) But if you're a reasonably active guy—if, for example, you can climb a flight of stairs without getting winded or do a couple of hours of yard work without alerting emergency medical technicians—you need to go a little harder than that.

There are many different formulas for figuring out how much aerobic exercise you need and how strenuously you should perform it. The American College of Sports Medicine recommends 30 minutes, three times week. For 20 minutes of each aerobic workout, you should be in your target heart-rate zone.

What the hell is that? Your target heart-rate zone is generally defined as 65 to 85 percent of your maximum heart rate. Your maximum can be determined a number of ways, but the easiest to remember is 220 minus your age. (That's accurate for only about 60 percent of the population—your real maximum could be higher or lower—but it gives you a ballpark estimate that's fine for most exercisers.)

So if you're 30 years old, your theoretical maximum heart rate is 190 (220 − 30 = 190). To calculate the lower end of your target zone, multiply your predicted maximum by 0.65 (190 × 0.65 = 123.5). Multiply your max by 0.85 to get the upper end of your target zone (190 × 0.85 = 161.5). When you start an aerobic workout, you can round off and remember the numbers 125 and 160, and that's close enough. Try to exercise hard enough to get your heart rate up into that zone.

There are three ways to know if you're in the zone.

1. Wear a heart-rate monitor.
2. Go to a gym and use the hand grips on high-end aerobic machines, which tell you your heart rate after you grip them for a few seconds.
3. Count your heartbeats at your wrist or neck for 10 seconds, and multiply by six. So let's say you're the 30-year-old in the example we've been using: If you put your fingers on your wrist in the middle of aerobic exercise and count 21 beats in 10 seconds, you're in the low end of your target zone (21 × 6 = 126). If you count 26 beats in 10 seconds, you're at the high end (26 × 6 = 156).

## THE LEVEL-ONE AEROBIC CHALLENGE

When you're just starting an aerobic exercise program, you don't need to spend a full 20 minutes in your target heart-rate zone. You can do the majority of your workout at an easy pace that's below what it would take to get your heart up to its target zone. If you can get into your target heart-rate zone with a brisk walk, a slower walk will work fine. If you need to jog to get your heart rate up to its target zone, a brisk walk may be an ideal easy-pace exercise.

In Week 2 of Level One (or in both weeks, if you feel up to it) you should do three aerobic workouts, giving yourself a day's rest between workouts. Do a total of 15 minutes of exercise in each workout, broken down as follows:

- 5 minutes at easy pace
- 5 minutes at target pace
- 5 minutes at easy pace

## EATING ESSENTIALS:
# THE TRUTH ABOUT FOOD

High-protein diets must be good, because your coworker lost 27 pounds in a month while following one. Low-fat diets also must be good, because on TV some skinny guy with a weird-looking mustache said they are. Then there was that news report explaining that if you have Syndrome X, a high-carbohydrate diet could lead to diabetes and heart disease. And everyone knows that sugar makes you fat. But what did that newspaper say about the Mediterranean Diet? We're supposed to eat olive oil, right? But isn't olive oil a fat, and didn't the skinny guy on TV say not to eat fat?

The only way you could avoid becoming confused about food today is if you never watched TV, read, or talked to anyone. If you tried to incorporate all the nutrition information floating around in the ether, either you'd eat everything (because there's someone out there to champion just about every food imaginable) or you'd eat nothing (because at one time or another every food has been demonized by a fad diet or nutrition guru).

In this stage of the Core Program, call a moratorium on all conflicting nutrition information and focus on the following simple rules.

**There are no bad foods.** Sure, there are foods that will kill you if you eat them every day in sufficient quantities to clog your arteries. But you know what? Having a little treat here or there won't have much effect on you one way or the other (unless it's poisoned, but that's a different issue). So forget everything you've heard about red meat, pasta, pizza, sugar, chocolate . . . any food that anyone has told you never to eat. You can get away with eating anything on occasion, in small quantities.

**There are no magic foods.** Just as there are no evil foods, neither is there one food that will turn around your life or, more to the point, your waistline. All foods have calories, so there's nothing you can eat in mass quantities without gaining weight. (Although, having said that, I'll concede that you are less likely to gain weight if your diet is filled with fruits and vegetables. Especially with all that extra time in the bathroom.)

**Diets don't work.** People who go on radical diets may lose weight fast, but they gain it all back—and more—when they go off the diets. Therefore, the net effect of most diets for most people is weight gain. To successfully manage your weight—to maintain it or lose the excess—you need to learn where you can permanently cut calories without feeling hungry or deprived.

## SIMPLE WAYS TO CUT CALORIES

Though almost everyone eats some of the following foods sometimes, lean people don't eat them very often: bacon; café latte made with whole milk; cream cheese; doughnuts; fast-food hamburgers, breakfast sandwiches, or fried-chicken or -fish sandwiches; french fries; hot dogs; onion rings; pastries; potato chips; and sausage. These foods are mostly fat, with little protein for muscle-building, carbohydrates for energy, or vitamins and minerals for health and vitality. They're poor choices when you want to maximize muscle and minimize flab.

If one of these is your favorite food, don't despair. We're not saying that you should never eat it again—remember, there are no bad foods. We just want you to realize that you can't eat it every day and still achieve the abs you want. Treat it like the delicacy that it is, saving it for special occasions. And when you do eat it, don't just gulp it down. Instead, really savor it.

Though no food has magic qualities

## THE REPLACEMENT PLAYERS

Besides rationing certain foods to cut calories, you can also reduce your caloric intake by making substitutions. Many foods have equivalents that taste about the same but have fewer calories. Here are some examples of high-calorie foods and their lower-calorie taste-alikes.

| INSTEAD OF. . . | TRY. . . |
| --- | --- |
| Prime rib | Sirloin |
| Full-fat mayonnaise | Low-fat or nonfat mayo |
| Baby Ruth, Snickers, or Reese's Peanut Butter Cup | Milky Way, Butterfinger, or 3 Musketeers |
| Pancakes topped with syrup | Pancakes topped with low-fat vanilla yogurt |
| Ritz Crackers | Stoned Wheat Thins |
| 1 Hostess Fruit Pie | 2 Hostess Twinkies |
| Granola bar | Cereal bar |
| Ready-to-eat popcorn | Tortilla chips |

that will change your life, here are some that are packed with high quantities of the most worthy nutrients: artichokes, beans, beets, black or green tea, blueberries, bran, broccoli, brown rice, brussels sprouts, cabbage, cantaloupe, carrots, cauliflower, chicken breasts, citrus fruit, eggs, fish, garlic, kale, kiwifruit, mangoes, milk, mi- take and shiitake mushrooms, nectarines, oatmeal, olive oil, onions, papayas, peas, peppers, prunes, salsa, spinach, sweet potatoes, tofu, and tomato products. If you eat more of these foods and fewer of the less-healthful ones listed earlier, you'll automatically reduce your calorie consumption.

## A WORD ABOUT WATER

Anything good quickly gets reduced to a cliché. Nutritionists began recommending that people drink at least eight 8-ounce glasses of water daily, and next thing you know, everyone in the gym is carrying a water bottle the size of a surface-to-air missile. In fact, doctors have even identified a new condition called dilutional hyponatremia, in which runners who drink too much water drain their bodies of essential nutrients.

But before the cliché, there was a problem. People were steadily dehydrating themselves with steady intakes of coffee and other caffeinated drinks like Mountain Dew during the day and with beer and wine at night. Sure, they were drinking plenty of beverages, but the beverages they were drinking had a diuretic effect. You've heard the expression that you don't buy beer, you only rent it? The same goes for all those diet colas and double mocha cappuccinos. They not only run right through you but also cause you to lose some of the water that was already in your system.

When you become dehydrated, you lose muscle strength since water is a huge component of muscle. You also lose muscle control since the nerves that coordinate your muscles depend on water to help them work efficiently.

You need to lose 2 percent of your body's weight in water before you start to feel thirsty. (That is, if you weigh 200 pounds, you'll lose 4 pounds of water before your body tells you to hit the water fountain.) But by the time you've lost that much water, you may already have sacrificed one-fifth of your strength and half of your aerobic power.

Each morning, fill a 1-liter bottle with water. Drink it all by the end of the day. Along with the other liquids you take in—such as milk, juices, and soups—that should be plenty of water to keep your body running smoothly.

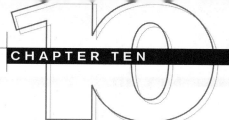

# CHAPTER TEN

# ESSENTIAL PROGRESS
## LEVEL TWO

**N**ow you're going to turn up the volume a little bit. Here's what Level Two will ask you to do.

- Increase your ab workout from three abdominal exercises to six, along with a more advanced lower-back exercise.
- Ramp up your aerobic exercise from 15 minutes a session to 24 minutes in Week 3, then 28 minutes in Week 4.
- Examine the nutrient content of the foods in your diet, and strive to balance the carbohydrates, protein, and fat.

## THE LEVEL-TWO ROUTINE

- Do this routine three times a week.
- Do one set of each exercise.
- Do 12 repetitions of each exercise and work up to 14 the first week. The next week, start with 16 reps of each and work up to 18.
- Push yourself a little harder. When you feel that you're finished with an exercise, try to gut out one more repetition, if you can do it with good form.
- Rest for fewer than 5 seconds between exercises.

**BENEFITS**
OF LEVEL TWO

Increased strength and endurance in your abdominal and lower-back muscles

Improved aerobic endurance

Weight loss from increased exercise

More energy from your higher fitness level and balanced diet

# Hip Up

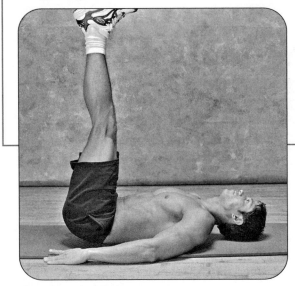
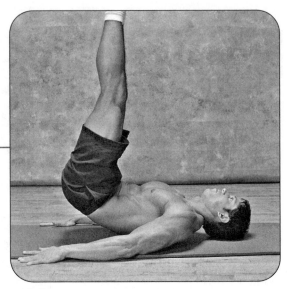

**READY, SET:**

Lie on your back with your legs raised directly over your hips; your knees should be slightly bent. Place your hands palms-down at your sides for support, and relax your head and neck.

**GO:**

Use your lower abs to raise your hips off the floor and toward your rib cage, elevating your feet straight up toward the ceiling. Hold for a second.

Then, in a controlled motion, slowly lower your hips back to the starting position. As they lightly touch the floor, repeat.

## PERFORMANCE TIPS

■ Don't kick with your legs to help elevate your hips; make your lower abs do the work.

■ Use your hands for stability, not to press your hips upward.

■ Try to pause at the top of the movement. It'll be difficult, but the longer you can hold this position, the better a contraction you'll get in your lower ab muscles.

# Reverse Crunch

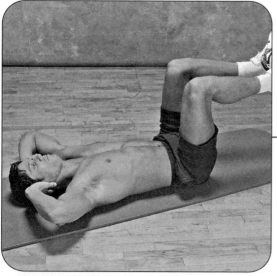

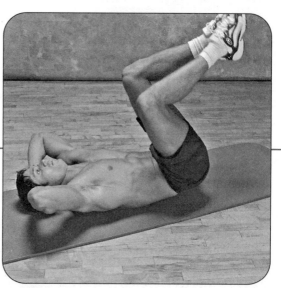

## READY, SET:

Lie on your back with your head and neck relaxed and your hands behind your ears. You want your lower body to form two right angles: Your thighs should be perpendicular to your upper body, with your lower legs parallel to the floor.

## GO:

Use your lower abs to raise your hips off the floor and toward your rib cage.

Then, in a controlled motion, slowly lower your hips back to the starting position. As they lightly touch the floor, repeat.

## PERFORMANCE TIPS

- Make sure your lower abs do the work. If you rock up and down, you're using momentum to aid you in the exercise, taking work away from your lower abs.

- Don't rest your hips on the floor at the bottom of the movement or let your lower legs drop down.

- Keep constant tension on your abs.

- Use your hands for balance. Don't use them to push off.

- Keep your head and neck relaxed.

# Crossover

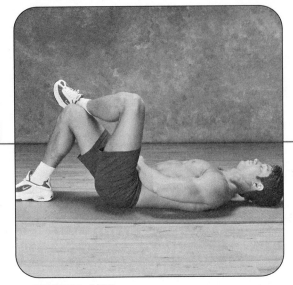 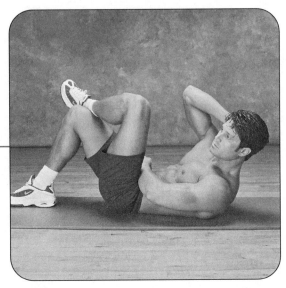

### READY, SET:

Lie on your back with your knees up and your feet on the floor. Cross your left leg over your right leg. Your left ankle should rest just below your right knee, making a triangle between your legs. Put your right hand behind your head, with your elbow extended to the side. Rest your head and elbow on the floor. Place your left hand on your right obliques or at your left side.

### GO:

Use your right obliques to raise your right shoulder and cross it toward your left knee.

Then, in a controlled motion, slowly lower your shoulder back to the starting position. As soon as your shoulder blade lightly touches the floor, repeat.

When you finish all of your repetitions on your right side, switch positions to work your left side: Put your right ankle below your left knee, put your left hand behind your head, and raise your left shoulder toward your right knee. Do the same number of reps on your left side.

## PERFORMANCE TIPS

■ Make sure that your entire torso twists up and toward your knee. Don't just move your elbow or shoulder. Don't move your knee toward your shoulder.

■ Feel the squeeze in your oblique muscles on the side that you're working. You'll probably also feel it in your upper abs on that side, which is fine.

■ Don't rest at the bottom of the movement; keep constant tension on your abs.

# Oblique Crunch

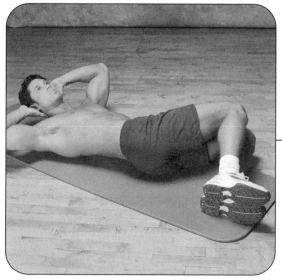

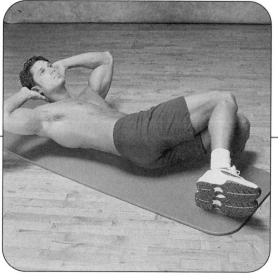

## READY, SET:

Lie on your back with your knees up, and let your legs fall to the left. Keep your shoulders flat on the floor. Keep your head and neck relaxed, with your hands behind your ears.

## GO:

Use your right obliques to raise your rib cage toward your pelvis and lift your shoulder blades off the floor. Hold for a second.

Then, in a controlled motion, slowly lower your shoulders back to the starting position. As soon as your shoulder blades lightly touch the floor, repeat.

When you finish all of your repetitions on your right side, switch positions to work your left side. Do the same number of reps on your left side.

## PERFORMANCE TIPS

■ If your top leg won't go all the way down when you let your legs fall to the side, let it rest in a comfortable position as close to your bottom leg as possible.

■ Try to keep your shoulders parallel or as close to parallel to the floor as possible.

■ You should feel the contraction in your rectus abdominis and in your obliques on the side that you're working.

■ As you get tired, you'll tend to lead off the movement by lifting a single shoulder off the floor. Focus on starting the movement with your abdominals and getting both shoulders off the floor.

# Crunch: Legs Up

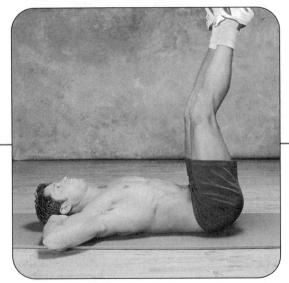

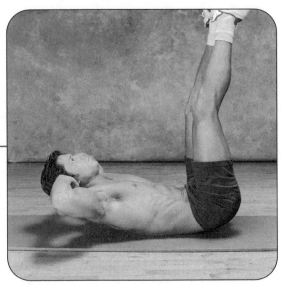

### READY, SET:

Lie on your back with your legs raised directly over your hips; your knees should be slightly bent. Keep your head and neck relaxed, with your hands behind your ears.

### GO:

Use your upper abs to raise your rib cage toward your pelvis and lift your shoulder blades off the floor. Hold for a second.

Then, in a controlled motion, slowly lower your shoulders back to the starting position. As soon as your shoulder blades lightly touch the floor, repeat.

## PERFORMANCE TIPS

■ Look up toward your feet on each repetition.

■ If you have problems holding your legs perpendicular to your upper body, you can rest them against a wall. That makes the exercise a little easier, so do this for only a workout or two, until you can hold your legs up without support.

# Crunch: Feet Flat

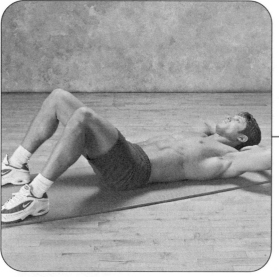 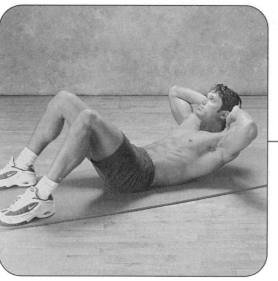

### READY, SET:

Lie on your back with your knees bent, your feet flat on the floor, your head and neck relaxed, and your hands behind your ears.

### GO:

Use your upper abs to raise your rib cage toward your pelvis and lift your shoulder blades off the floor. Hold for a second.

Then, in a controlled motion, slowly lower your shoulders back to the starting position. As soon as your shoulder blades lightly touch the floor, repeat.

## PERFORMANCE TIPS

■ Make sure your shoulder blades come off the floor each time. Don't just move your head and neck.

■ Move up and down slowly; don't use momentum to finish your repetitions.

■ Keep constant tension on your abs throughout the movement—don't rest at the bottom of the movement.

■ Pause at the top of the movement, after you've exhaled, and feel the squeeze go deeper into your abdominals.

# Superman

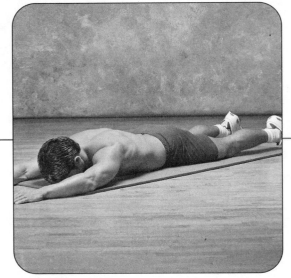
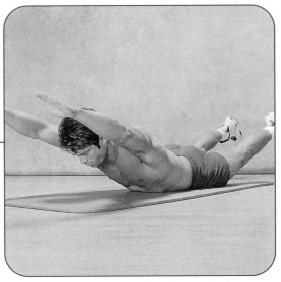

### READY, SET:

Lie facedown on the floor with your arms and legs extended and angled out slightly. Your palms should face the floor.

### GO:

Lift your arms and legs off the floor as if you were Superman flying. Hold for 3 seconds.

Then, in a controlled motion, slowly lower your arms and legs back to the starting position. As they lightly touch the floor, repeat.

## PERFORMANCE TIPS

■ Your head and neck will also rise off the floor on this exercise, but don't allow your neck to hyperextend backward. Keep your neck in line with your shoulders throughout the exercise. However much your shoulders rise, that's how high your neck should lift.

■ As in the lower-back exercise in Level One (the opposite arm and leg raise), you'll feel a contraction in your gluteals and hamstrings too.

■ If you can hold each contraction for longer than 3 seconds, do so. The more endurance you build in your lower back, the more improvements you'll feel in your posture.

■ Why don't I see any change in my stomach yet?

**This question requires a two-part answer.**

**First, you're building muscles with these abdominal exercises, and you probably won't see actual changes in them until after 6 weeks of the Core Program. That's just the way muscles work. Your strength and endurance will increase rapidly—you've probably already noticed this—but the muscle fibers won't actually get bigger until 6 to 8 weeks have passed.**

**Second, you probably haven't yet done much to reduce the fat around your midsection. As you increase your aerobic exercise and improve your eating habits, you'll see the fat start to disappear.**

■ The new Level-Two exercises are a lot tougher than the ones that carry over from Level One. Can't I just continue to do the Level-One exercises only for a while longer?

**I'll concede that the new Level-Two exercises are harder than those that you learned in Level One. But that's the nature of muscle building. You have to keep finding new ways to challenge your muscles, or they won't develop. In fact, the muscles can even go backward. If you keep doing the same old stuff the same old way, your body will get so good at it that it'll start using fewer muscle fibers to do the exercises, and you'll start to lose what you worked so hard to gain.**

**New challenges can be implemented in a variety of ways: by adding weight, increasing sets, decreasing rest time, changing the order of the exercises, and changing the exercises or adding new ones. Don't worry, we built in all these variations for you when we created the Core Program.**

■ I feel a little tug in my lower back when I do exercises like crossovers and oblique crunches. Is there a modification I can make?

**Do the exercises with a limited range of motion. That is, stop short of the point at which you feel a tug. Then, after your abdominal exercises, do the stretching exercises in chapter 6. Eventually, you should develop enough lower-back flexibility to do these exercises as described.**

**AEROBIC ESSENTIALS:**
# TURN UP THE VOLUME

Now it's time to put in some miles. In Level Two, you should increase both the time you spend in your target heart-rate zone and the total time you spend doing aerobic exercise. You'll start feeling different during Level Two. First, the increased volume of exercise should start to whittle down your waist a bit. Second, you should notice that you sleep better at night—if for no other reason than because you're more tired when you go to bed on the days in which you exercise—and feel more energetic the next day. It's a healthy cycle: Sleep better, have more energy. Can you handle that?

Here's the plan for Week 3. On 3 non-consecutive days this week, do this 24-minute aerobic workout.

- 5 minutes at easy pace
- 6 minutes at target pace
- 2 minutes at easy pace
- 6 minutes at target pace
- 5 minutes at easy pace

In Week 4, increase to the following 28-minute workout on each of your 3 aerobic days.

- 5 minutes at easy pace
- 8 minutes at target pace
- 2 minutes at easy pace
- 8 minutes at target pace
- 5 minutes at easy pace

## HOW TO HIT YOUR TARGET

Level One told you about the benefits of simple aerobic exercises like walking, jogging, cycling, and swimming. Those are still the best exercises for Level Two, but now you have to develop strategies for turning the volume up and down so you can quickly reach your target heart-rate zone, stay there for the required number of minutes, and then throttle down to give your body a break.

Here are a few options.

**Walk/jog.** Walk for the first 5 minutes. Around the 3-minute mark, start walking faster, feeling your breathing speeding up. Pump your arms to help you build up speed. After this 5-minute warmup, start jogging to get to your target pace. Walk again when it's time to go easy and for your cooldown at the end.

**Cycle easy/cycle hard.** On a bike, going from an easy pace to your target pace can be accomplished two ways: by pedaling faster or by pedaling in a higher gear. Or you can do a combination.

**Breaststroke/freestyle.** When swimming, you can warm up with the breaststroke for the first few laps, then hit your target pace with the freestyle stroke (also known as the crawl).

**Aerobic machines.** Of course, machines are great for taking the guesswork out of aerobic exercise. You don't get the fresh air (or, as in the case of the pool, that sinus-clearing chlorine aroma), but you do get a device that makes it easy to increase or decrease the intensity of the exercise. Push a button, and the machine goes faster, slopes higher (in the case of the treadmill), or makes you pedal harder (in the case of the stationary bike).

Best of all, machines free you from jogging in place at stoplights, from the worry of dodging traffic while changing gears, from wearing multiple layers of spandex in the dead of winter, and from plowing into the slower swimmers clogging your lane.

## EATING ESSENTIALS:
## KNOW WHAT'S ON YOUR FORK

Food has three macronutrients, or components: carbohydrates, protein, and fat. Science has understood what each is and does for a long time, but the proper balance of each in your diet has probably never been more controversial than as in the opening years of the 21st century.

Let's take a closer look at each of these macronutrients to help you develop a simple strategy for sufficient amounts of each in your diet.

## Protein

**Its essential function:** This amino acid builds and repairs muscles.

**The debate:** Serious weight lifters believe that to build the muscle they want, they need huge amounts of protein—typically double or even triple the amounts recommended for the general population.

Some diet gurus recommend huge protein intakes, probably because it's very hard for your body to convert protein to fat. It can use protein as energy, but that's hard too. It's the path of the greatest resistance, so excess protein is most often simply excreted—literally flushed down the toilet.

Nutritionists, on the other hand, tend to believe that almost everyone eats too much protein and that this protein is often in the form of high-fat foods like hamburgers, cheese, creamy sauces, and eggs.

**The truth (as of now):** If you exercise a lot—and particularly if you do a lot of resistance exercise—your body can use between 7 and 10 grams of protein per every 10 pounds of body weight, per day.

The best way to meet your protein requirement is through a combination of lean meats, fish, eggs, beans, and low-fat dairy products. But, if you're busy—for example, if you work in an office where you don't have access to healthy, low-fat, high-protein foods—you can turn to protein bars and shakes. There's nothing magical about the protein in supplements, no matter what the labels on the products tell you, but they work fine as food substitutes.

## Fat

**Its essential function:** Fat regulates your body temperature; protects your internal organs; helps your body use crucial nutrients like vitamin E, which protects cells from environmental damage; regulates your body's hormones, like testosterone; and provides energy that you use throughout the day.

**The debate:** One of the most cherished assumptions about weight loss is that eating fat makes you fat. This makes sense, considering that a gram of fat has about 9 calories, whereas a gram of protein or carbohydrate has just 4. A carbohydrate- or protein-rich food has fewer calories than the same amount of a fatty food, and thus it should be less likely to make you fatter.

But Americans tend to replace the fat in

## PROTEIN REPORT CARD

| FOOD | SERVING SIZE | AMOUNT OF PROTEIN (G) |
|---|---|---|
| Tuna | 6.5 oz can | 45.0 |
| Chicken breast | 4 oz | 36.0 |
| Refried beans | 1 cup | 15.0 |
| Broccoli, cooked | 1 cup | 5.8 |
| Whole-wheat bread | 2 slices | 4.8 |

their diets with larger quantities of high-carbohydrate foods, not equal quantities, and steadily get fatter instead of slimmer.

Worse, research has found that low-fat, high-carbohydrate diets could be deadly for people with the combination of diseases called Syndrome X. Other studies found that people eating a high-fat Mediterranean diet were actually healthier than Americans eating lower-fat diets.

**The truth (as of now):** You need fat in your diet. Besides performing important duties in your body, fat makes you feel fuller and more satisfied than you would if you ate meals without it.

But you have to distinguish between the three different kinds of fat. *Monounsaturated fats* are found in nuts, seeds, avocados, olives, wheat germ, and oils such as peanut, olive, canola, and flaxseed. These are the fats in the Mediterranean diet, and they have been shown to actually raise your body's good cholesterol (HDL, which reduces your risk of heart disease) and lower its bad cholesterol (LDL) without raising your total cholesterol.

*Polyunsaturated fats* include those in cold-water fish, like salmon, and in oils such as corn, safflower, and sesame. These also lower your risk of heart disease, particularly by lowering your levels of very low density lipoproteins (VLDL), the most dangerous type of cholesterol.

*Saturated fats* are found in eggs, meats, dairy products, shortening and lard, and coconut, palm, and palm kernel oils. There's not much good news about saturated fats. One important study found that the people who ate the most saturated fats had the highest rates of heart disease. Men in Finland who got 22.7 percent of their total calories from saturated fats had a 28.8 percent death rate from heart disease. Conversely, men in Japan who got just 3.8 percent of their calories from saturated fats had a minuscule 4.5 percent death rate from heart disease.

Your goal is to cut the saturated fats in your diet and increase the two types of unsaturated fats. Here are some suggestions about how to do that.

- Choose lower-fat dairy products and leaner cuts of meat.
- Eat more fish—a good goal is to eat at least two servings a week.
- Cook with small amounts of oil instead of butter, margarine, or shortening.

## Carbohydrates

**Their essential function:** Carbs are your body's preferred source of fuel.

**The debate:** Since it's so easy for your body to use carbohydrates for energy,

## FAT REPORT CARD

| FOOD | SERVING SIZE | AMOUNT OF FAT (G) |
|------|--------------|-------------------|
| Roast beef sandwich | 1 sandwich | 13.8 |
| Scrambled egg | 1 egg | 7.3 |
| Plain doughnut | 1 doughnut | 10.8 |
| Pork sausage | 1 link | 1.6 |
| Cheddar cheese | 1 oz | 9.0 |

nutritionists got the idea that carbs should make up the majority of your daily calories.

The problem is that the carbohydrates of choice tend to be easy-to-overeat breads, cereals, and baked goods. As has been discovered by anyone who has consumed an entire package of low-fat cookies when he meant to eat just one or two, these types of carbs just aren't very satisfying foods. So instead of eating a single bagel, people either eat two or stick with one but slather it in high-fat cream cheese.

Then the public figured out that carbohydrates can make the body hold on to excess water, which is something that serious bodybuilders have known for years. If you cut the carbs out of your diet, you immediately lose a few pounds of retained water and instantly look slimmer. But people who have tried super low carbohydrate diets find that these plans aren't sustainable. When the dieters go back to eating carbs, they quickly bloat back up and generally end up weighing more than they did before they started their diets.

**The truth (as of now):** Carbohydrates don't make you fat, but they can lead to overeating if you eat the wrong kinds and eat them exclusively, without fat and protein to help you feel fuller faster.

The key is to eat more complex than simple carbohydrates, or at least the right kind of simple carbs. Here's how to tell the difference.

*Complex carbohydrates* are absorbed more slowly by your body, giving you a steady energy flow. These include vegetables, whole-grain breads and cereals (including oatmeal), beans, and pasta.

*Simple carbohydrates* are quickly digested. These include dairy products (the carbohydrate source is called lactose), fruits and fruit juices (fructose), and honey, syrup, and table sugar (sucrose). As a rule, dairy products and fruits are good for you and should be included in your diet. But it's the sucrose calories in sweets that cause spikes and crashes in energy levels.

## A LITTLE EXPERIMENT

Here are several ways to ensure that you include all the right types of macronutrients in your meals and don't overeat.

- Divide your plate into halves: half carbohydrate-rich foods, half protein- and fat-rich foods. This is a crude and completely unscientific way to get enough protein while limiting the foods that you might tend to overeat. But, on the bright side, it's easy to remember and easy to implement.
- Make sure your food doesn't touch the edges of the plate or the other foods on the plate. This helps you limit portion sizes.
- After you eat your plate of food, wait for a half-hour. If you're still hungry, eat more. But chances are, you'll decide that you feel satiated and wait until your next meal before eating again. This cuts down on impulse eating—that is, gobbling down large quantities of food just because you're used to eating that much.

# CHAPTER ELEVEN

# ESSENTIAL ACHIEVEMENT
## LEVEL THREE

This third level asks more of you, but by the time you complete it, you will be able to see a difference in your abs. Here are the specifics of what you'll do in Level Three.

- Perform nine abdominal exercises and one lower-back exercise.
- Increase your aerobic exercise to 30 minutes, three times a week, including 20 minutes in your target heart-rate zone.
- Eat enough protein to facilitate muscle building.

## THE LEVEL-THREE ROUTINE

- Learn three new ab exercises, plus a back extension.
- Perform the workout four times a week until you are able to complete the designated number of repetitions of each exercise.
- Do one set of each exercise.
- Start with 12 repetitions of each ab exercise, and increase your reps by one by your fourth workout of the week. The next week, start with 14 reps of each, and work up to 15 of each.
- Rest for 5 to 30 seconds between exercises.

If any of the exercises is too difficult, repeat the Level-Two exercise that works the same ab area, but increase to the number of repetitions recommended here.

---

**BENEFITS**
OF LEVEL THREE

A very high level of strength and endurance in your abdominal muscles, with the possibility of new muscle mass becoming visible at this stage

Increased efficiency of your heart and lungs from aerobic exercise

Accelerated weight loss from the higher volume of exercise

# Corkscrew

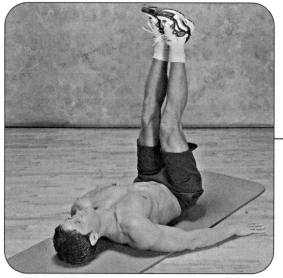

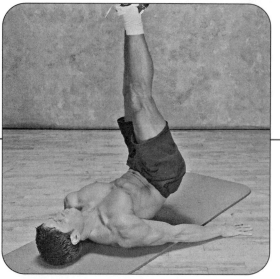

## READY, SET:

Lie on your back with your legs raised directly over your hips; your knees should be slightly bent. Place your hands palms-down at your sides for support, and relax your head and neck.

## GO:

Use your lower abs to raise your hips off the floor and toward your rib cage, elevating your feet straight up toward the ceiling. Simultaneously twist your hips to the right in a corkscrew motion. Hold for a second.

Then, in a controlled motion, slowly lower yourself back to the starting position. As soon as your hips lightly touch the floor, raise them again, and this time twist them to the left. That's one repetition.

## PERFORMANCE TIPS

■ Each workout, switch the side on which you start: If you twist to the right and then to the left in the first workout, reverse that order and start with a twist to the left the next time you do corkscrews.

■ Pause at the top of the movement.

■ Don't kick up with your legs to elevate your hips; keep the movement controlled, even if you must stop before you reach the suggested number of reps.

■ Use your hands for stability, not to press your hips upward.

# Hip Up

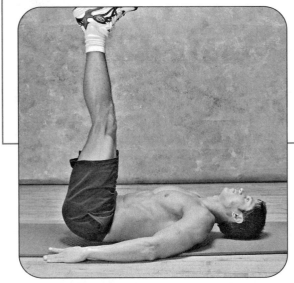 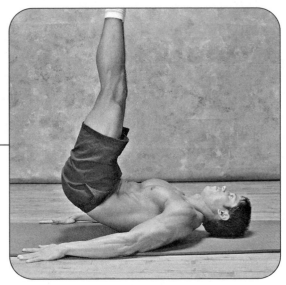

**READY, SET:**

Lie on your back with your legs raised directly over your hips; your knees should be slightly bent. Place your hands palms-down at your sides for support, and relax your head and neck.

**GO:**

Use your lower abs to raise your hips off the floor and toward your rib cage, elevating your feet straight up toward the ceiling. Hold for a second.

Then, in a controlled motion, slowly lower your hips back to the starting position. As they lightly touch the floor, repeat.

## PERFORMANCE TIPS

■ Don't kick with your legs to help elevate your hips; make your lower abs do the work.

■ Use your hands for stability, not to press your hips upward.

■ Try to pause at the top of the movement. It'll be difficult, but the longer you can hold this position, the better a contraction you'll get in your lower ab muscles.

# Reverse Crunch

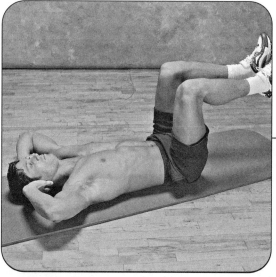

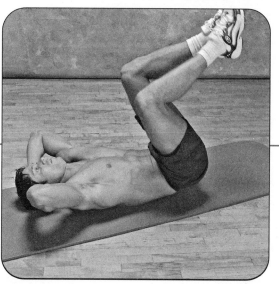

### READY, SET:

Lie on your back with your head and neck relaxed and your hands behind your ears. You want your lower body to form two right angles: Your thighs should be perpendicular to your upper body, with your lower legs parallel to the floor.

### GO:

Use your lower abs to raise your hips off the floor and toward your rib cage.

Then, in a controlled motion, slowly lower your hips back to the starting position. As they lightly touch the floor, repeat.

## PERFORMANCE TIPS

■ Make sure your lower abs do the work. If you rock up and down, you're using momentum to aid you in the exercise, taking work away from your lower abs.

■ Don't rest your hips on the floor at the bottom of the movement or let your lower legs drop down.

■ Keep constant tension on your abs.

■ Use your hands for balance. Don't use them to push off.

■ Keep your head and neck relaxed.

# Crossover

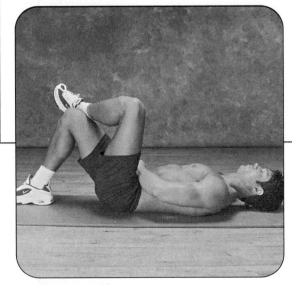 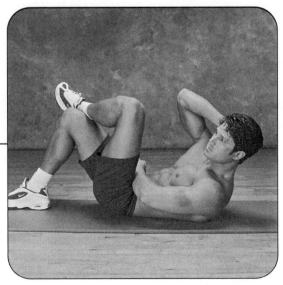

## READY, SET:

Lie on your back with your knees up and your feet on the floor. Cross your left leg over your right leg. Your left ankle should rest just below your right knee, making a triangle between your legs. Put your right hand behind your head, with your elbow extended to the side. Rest your head and elbow on the floor. Place your left hand on your right obliques or at your left side.

## GO:

Use your right obliques to raise your right shoulder and cross it toward your left knee.

Then, in a controlled motion, slowly lower your shoulder back to the starting position. As soon as your shoulder blade lightly touches the floor, repeat.

When you finish all of your repetitions on your right side, switch positions to work your left side: Put your right ankle below your left knee, put your left hand behind your head, and raise your left shoulder toward your right knee. Do the same number of reps on your left side.

## PERFORMANCE TIPS

■ Make sure that your entire torso twists up and toward your knee. Don't just move your elbow or shoulder. Don't move your knee toward your shoulder.

■ Feel the squeeze in your oblique muscles on the side that you're working. You'll probably also feel it in your upper abs on that side, which is fine.

■ Don't rest at the bottom of the movement; keep constant tension on your abs.

# Oblique Crunch

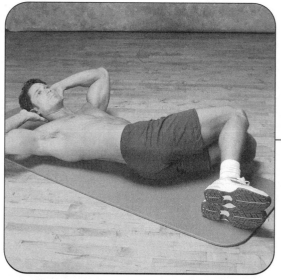 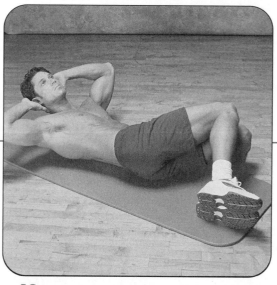

### READY, SET:

Lie on your back with your knees up, and let your legs fall to the left. Keep your shoulders flat on the floor. Keep your head and neck relaxed, with your hands behind your ears.

### GO:

Use your right obliques to raise your rib cage toward your pelvis and lift your shoulder blades off the floor. Hold for a second.

Then, in a controlled motion, slowly lower your shoulders back to the starting position. As soon as your shoulder blades lightly touch the floor, repeat.

When you finish all of your repetitions on your right side, switch positions to work your left side. Do the same number of reps on your left side.

## PERFORMANCE TIPS

- If your top leg won't go all the way down when you let your legs fall to the side, let it rest in a comfortable position as close to your bottom leg as possible.

- Try to keep your shoulders parallel or as close to parallel to the floor as possible.

- You should feel the contraction in your rectus abdominis and in your obliques on the side that you're working.

- As you get tired, you'll tend to lead off the movement by lifting a single shoulder off the floor. Focus on starting the movement with your abdominals and getting both shoulders off the floor.

# Catch

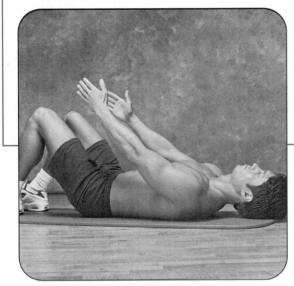 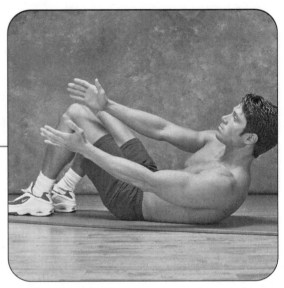

## READY, SET:

Lie on your back with your knees bent, your feet flat on the floor, and your hands extended toward your knees.

## GO:

Use your ab muscles to raise your torso on a diagonal line, lifting your right shoulder toward your left knee and reaching both hands above and to the outside of your left knee as if you were going to catch a ball that was being thrown to you. Hold for a second.

Then, in a controlled motion, slowly lower your shoulder back to the starting position. As soon as your shoulder blade lightly touches the floor, do the movement to your right side, lifting your left shoulder toward your right knee. That's one repetition.

## PERFORMANCE TIPS

■ Because you're trying to move your torso on a diagonal line, the contraction in your abdominals should feel different from the one you got with the crunches and crossovers that you've done in this program. That's the key to continued abdominal development—different angles, different contractions.

■ With your head completely unsupported, you may feel a little discomfort in your neck. You can try supporting it with one hand and reaching with the other hand.

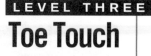
# Toe Touch

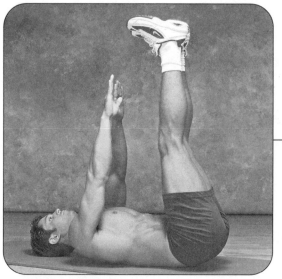

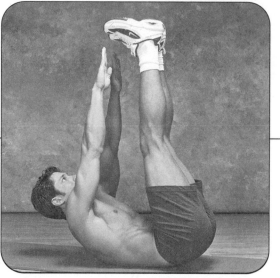

## READY, SET:

Lie on your back with your legs raised directly over your hips; your knees should be slightly bent. Raise your arms straight up, pointing toward your toes, and relax your head and neck.

## GO:

Use your upper abs to raise your rib cage toward your pelvis, lift your shoulder blades off the floor, and reach toward your toes. Hold for a second.

Then, in a controlled motion, slowly lower your shoulders back to the starting position. As soon as your shoulder blades lightly touch the floor, repeat.

## PERFORMANCE TIPS

■ You probably won't be able to touch your toes; just get as close as you can. Your range of motion will improve as you get used to the movement.

■ If you have problems holding your legs perpendicular to your upper body, you can rest them against a wall. Or have a training partner hold up your legs. You probably also want to work on your flexibility by doing the stretches in chapter 6.

■ A challenging variation is to reach to one side of your feet with your hands, making it an exercise for your obliques as well as your upper abs. If you try it, make sure you do an equal number of repetitions to each side.

# Crunch: Legs Up

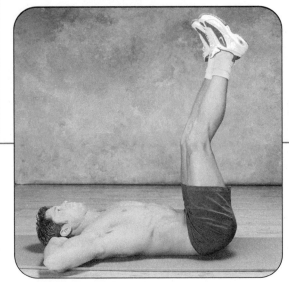 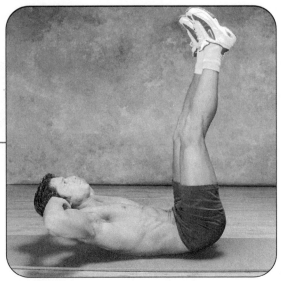

**READY, SET:**

Lie on your back with your legs raised directly over your hips; your knees should be slightly bent. Keep your head and neck relaxed, with your hands behind your ears.

**GO:**

Use your upper abs to raise your rib cage toward your pelvis and lift your shoulder blades off the floor. Hold for a second.

Then, in a controlled motion, slowly lower your shoulders back to the starting position. As soon as your shoulder blades lightly touch the floor, repeat.

## PERFORMANCE TIPS

■ Look up toward your feet on each repetition.

■ If you have problems holding your legs perpendicular to your upper body, you can rest them against a wall. That makes the exercise a little easier, so do this for only a workout or two, until you can hold your legs up without support.

# Crunch: Frog Legs

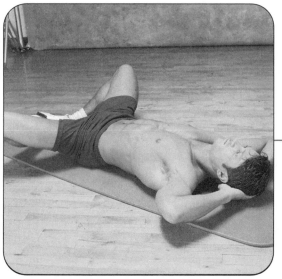

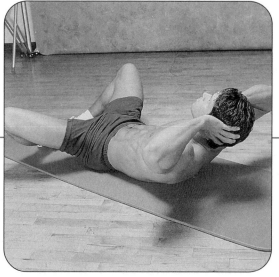

### READY, SET:

Lie on your back with your legs apart, your knees bent, and the soles of your feet together. Keep your head and neck relaxed, with your hands behind your ears.

### GO:

Use your upper abs to raise your rib cage toward your pelvis and lift your shoulder blades off the floor. Hold for a second.

Then, in a controlled motion, slowly lower your shoulders back to the starting position. As soon as your shoulder blades lightly touch the floor, repeat.

## PERFORMANCE TIPS

■ Keep a fist's distance between your chin and chest. As you get exhausted, it becomes very tempting to strain your head forward to start repetitions.

■ One trick to keep your chin from moving toward your chest is to focus your eyes straight up at a point on the ceiling.

■ This is a great exercise for feeling your abdominal muscles work. You may want to hold this contraction longer than you do on the other exercises— 2 to 5 seconds, instead of just 1 second.

# Isometric Back Extension

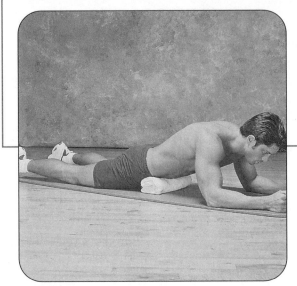

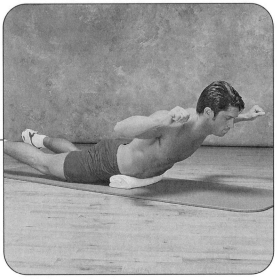

**READY, SET:**

Lie facedown on the floor with a rolled-up towel beneath your navel and your legs about shoulder-width apart. Lift your torso and rest your weight on your forearms, as if you were lying on the floor to watch TV.

**GO:**

Slowly lift your forearms off the floor and out to your sides while keeping your torso still. Hold for the count specified in the "Performance Tips."

Then, in a controlled motion, slowly lower your forearms back to the floor. Feel some of the tension release from your lower back, and repeat.

## PERFORMANCE TIPS

- The first time you do this exercise, start with four repetitions, holding each for 4 seconds. Add a rep each workout, until you can do six reps of 4 seconds each. Then, decrease to five reps, but hold each for 5 seconds. Work up to seven 5-second reps.

- If you have a strong lower back, you may need to hold for longer than the number of seconds recommended here to feel the exercise do its work.

- Keep your torso and neck in the same position throughout the exercise.

- Don't hold your breath. Breathe normally. You can even count the seconds of each contraction with your breathing, taking one strong breath per second.

## AEROBIC ESSENTIALS:
# GETTING RESULTS

Ready to go to the next stage? Good. In Level Three, your cardiovascular workouts are finally going to reach the standards suggested by the American College of Sports Medicine—at least 30 minutes, three times a week, including 20 minutes in your target heart-rate zone.

Here's your 32-minute program for Week 5 of the Core Program.

- 5 minutes at easy pace
- 10 minutes at target pace
- 2 minutes at easy pace
- 10 minutes at target pace
- 5 minutes at easy pace

By Week 6 at this level, you'll even do all 20 target-heart-rate minutes consecutively.

- 5 minutes at easy pace
- 20 minutes at target pace
- 5 minutes at easy pace

## RATING YOUR WORKOUT

When you do aerobic exercise, trying to figure your heart rate can get to be a pain in the neck (literally, if that's where you check your pulse). It breaks up the flow of your workout, and if you're riding a bike, it could lead to some nasty road rash.

Even if you use a heart-rate monitor, a lot of things can go wrong.

- Your sweat or electronic interference can cause bad readings.
- If you consumed caffeine or took an allergy medication containing ephedrine or pseudoephedrine be-

fore your workout, your heart rate could be artificially high.

- High heat or humidity can also raise your pulse rate.
- Some heart and blood pressure medications can make your heart rate artificially lower than it normally would be at your level of exertion.

Whether you're using a monitor or not, you could be one of the guys for whom the 220-minus-your-age formula isn't close to accurate in determining your maximum heart rate. As explained in the Level-One aerobics section, the formula is 100 percent accurate for only about 60 percent of the population. Among the other 40 percent of us, the actual maximum rate could be as much as 30 beats per minute higher or lower. So if you're 30 years old, the formula predicts that your maximum heart rate is 190 beats per minute. But your true max could actually be 160 or 220.

Don't worry, I wouldn't point out a problem without offering a solution. The easiest way to monitor your aerobic workout is with a method called perceived exertion, in which you rate how hard you're working on a scale from 1 to 10.

The table on page 89 shows the full perceived exertion scale. Here's how it works. In the Level-Three workouts, your goal is to get into the 4 to 5 range, or between somewhat hard and hard. Keep in mind, though, that this is a moving target. You can run the same route at the same speed three times in the same week, and each time it may feel like a different level of exertion—4 one day, 6 another, 5 on the third.

■ It seems that when I have a good workout, it's followed by a bad one.

I could fill an entire chapter with explanations of why a workout may not be as good as the one that preceded it. Here are some factors that may come into play.

**1.** You didn't eat enough before the workout, and your body is starving. That's a bad sign—your body will take protein from your muscles to use for energy.

Conversely, you may have eaten too soon before your workout. That's bad too; food could make you feel sluggish, and it could also interfere with your muscle-building hormones, diminishing the results of your workout.

A good rule is to eat protein and carbohydrates an hour or two before your workout and to try to avoid fat during that time.

**2.** You're under stress. Your body releases a hormone called cortisol in reaction to stress, and this neutralizes testos-terone, your main muscle-building hormone. (Cortisol also signals your body to store fat in your midsection, which negates the gains you make doing abdominal exercises.)

**3.** You didn't recuperate properly from your last workout. Let's say you walked into the gym on Monday and had one of your best workouts ever. Then you went back in on Wednesday and had a mediocre workout, doing fewer repetitions of most of your exercises. Your body could be telling you that it needed an extra day to recover. The older you are, the more likely it is that this will happen. If you're over 40, you may need to take 2 days off between muscle-building workouts.

Recuperation also involves sleeping well each night and eating consistently to give your body healthy, balanced meals throughout each day.

■ When my workouts get longer, I find that I zone out a little. I start thinking about what I'm having for dinner or what video I'm going to rent.

Everyone struggles with focus sometimes. One key to maintaining concentration is giving yourself a reason to get excited about each workout. That's one of the reasons why the Core Program includes new challenges each workout. You're always trying to do one more repetition on each exercise, and you add new exercises every 2 weeks.

You can apply this to any other type of workout you do. If you lift weights, make sure that you do more repetitions or use more weight on each exercise each time you do it. If you run, either try to do your usual route faster or take a new route altogether.

Have a new goal for each workout, and focus will most likely take care of itself. (And no, "I just want to get through this before I hit the drive-thru" doesn't count as a goal.)

| NUMBER RATING | DEGREE OF DIFFICULTY | RATE OF BREATHING | ABILITY TO TALK | % OF MAXIMUM AEROBIC CAPACITY |
|---|---|---|---|---|
| 1 | Very easy | Normal | Until someone interrupts | 35.0 |
| 2 | Easy | Still normal | Yak, yak, yak | 45.0 |
| 3 | Light, but starting to feel like exercise | Comfortable | No problem yet | 55.0 |
| 4 | Somewhat hard | Noticeably deeper | Possible, but no campaign speeches | 65.0 |
| 5 | Hard | Deep but steady | Just name, rank, and serial number | 75.0 |
| 6 | Between hard and very hard | Deep and getting faster | Name only | 85.0 |
| 7 | Very hard | Deep and fast | Initials only | 90.0 |
| 8 | Very, very hard | Very deep, very fast | Maybe a grunt | 95.0 |
| 9 | So hard you can do it for only a few seconds | Panting | A gasp | 97.5 |
| 10 | Maximum effort | Can't breathe | Can't even gasp | 100.0 |

That's okay. Your goal is to make sure that the exercise feels as hard as you want it to. You don't need to cover a certain amount of ground in a set time; leave that to the competitive athletes.

## BURNING BY NUMBERS

By now, you're probably wondering exactly what all this exercise adds up to—or, more accurately, what it subtracts from your waistline. You know that if you're trying to lose weight through exercise, the bottom line is how many calories you burn. Here's a formula to help you calculate the number of calories burned in an hour when you're engaged in certain common aerobic activities.

First, figure out your weight in kilograms by dividing your weight in pounds by 2.2. Then, multiply the result by the metabolic value assigned to your exercise activity in "The Value of Exercise" on page 90. The total is the number of calories you'll burn in an hour while participating in that activity.

| ACTIVITY | DEGREE OF DIFFICULTY | METABOLIC VALUE |
|---|---|---|
| Basketball | Pickup game | 8.0 |
| Bicycling | Easy (10–12 mph) | 6.0 |
| | Somewhat hard (12–14 mph) | 8.0 |
| | Hard (14–16 mph) | 10.0 |
| Running | Easy (10-min mile) | 8.0 |
| | Somewhat hard (8-min mile) | 12.5 |
| | Hard (6-min mile) | 16.0 |
| Soccer | Easy | 7.0 |
| | Hard | 10.0 |
| Swimming | Easy | 8.0 |
| | Hard | 10.0 |
| Tai chi or yoga | — | 4.0 |
| Tennis | — | 8.0 |
| Walking | Easy | 2.5 |
| | Somewhat hard | 3.5 |
| | Hard | 4.0 |

## EATING ESSENTIALS:
# FOOD FOR MUSCLE

Up to this point, it's been enough of a challenge for you to simply modify your food intake by making slightly better choices in what you eat, slimming down your portions, and eating balanced meals. But now you're going to add another level of difficulty: making sure you get enough protein.

Level Two of the Core Program told you to get between 7 and 10 grams of protein for every 10 pounds of body weight if you're trying to build muscle. To see if you're in this range, for one day, add up the grams of protein in all the foods you eat. You should be able to get the figures from food labels. When you eat out, you can estimate by writing down the foods you order and then checking their protein content in a book called *Bowes and Church's Food Values of Portions Commonly Used*. The title doesn't exactly trip off the tongue, but it's complete and easy to use, and your local library probably has it. If you go to a fast-food chain restaurant, you can usually go to the company's Web site to find the nutrition information. (While you're there, check out the fat content of what you just ate, and decide if you really want to make a return trip.)

## READING FOOD LABELS

Ideally, an ab-conscious guy like you would eat only healthful, whole foods like whole grains and fresh fruits and vegetables. But despite your ab-consciousness, you're still a guy, and it's unlikely that you'll completely strip processed foods from your diet.

So as part of your Core Program healthy-eating plan, you should start paying attention to the ingredients and Nutrition Facts labels on the packaged foods that you do eat. Here are some of the most important things to look out for when perusing those labels.

Ingredients are listed in order of weight. As a rule of thumb, you want to avoid foods that list a type of sugar first on the list (high-fructose corn syrup is often the chart topper).

The serving sizes are usually half of what you'll actually eat. A loaf of bread, for example, will tell you that a serving size is one slice. But when do you ever eat just one slice of bread? So, realistically, you have to double the serving size to figure out the nutritional value of what you're eating.

Another example is a can of soup. You know you're going to go home, dump it into a bowl, zap it in the microwave for a couple of minutes, and eat all of it. But when you look on the label, you see that one can is actually two servings. So whatever nutrients are listed—calories, fat, protein, and all the rest—have to be doubled.

Fat is often replaced by sugar. When you get tempted by the words *reduced fat*, *low-fat*, or *fat-free* on a package, a quick scan of the label will show you that the slimmed-down food is also sugared up. (And you should also know that reduced fat means the product has 25 percent less fat than the regular version, which is not much help when you're talking about something that's virtually all fat to begin with, like bacon.)

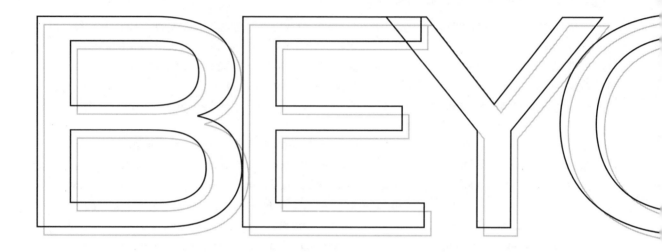

OND

THE CORE

PROGRAM

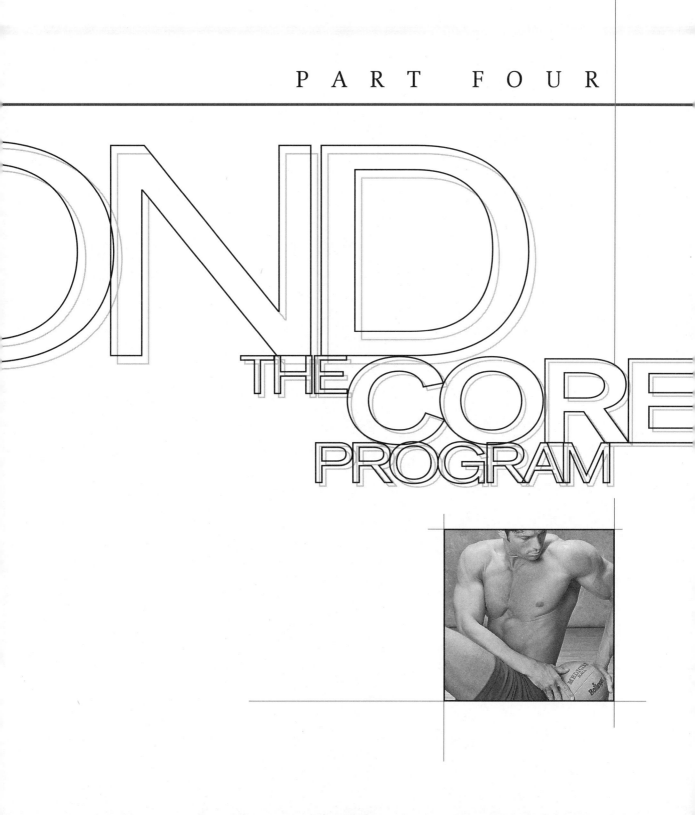

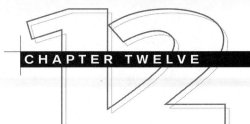

# CHAPTER TWELVE

# ESSENTIAL MAINTENANCE

**Y**our abs are toned and starting to feel hard. You can probably see the ridges developing around the top and sides of your abdomen. Meanwhile, your posture is more upright, your energy level is higher, your weight is probably lower, and you sleep longer and deeper.

Best of all, you're just getting started. What you can do in 6 weeks is just a small fraction of what you can accomplish with years of steady exercise, smart eating, and healthy living.

So what exactly are you going to do for the rest of your life? These guidelines will help you continue the process you've successfully begun.

## ABDOMINAL EXERCISE

You don't want to add any more ab exercises than you're doing now—nine are enough. Your goal is to make the exercises you do progressively tougher. Here's how.

■ Increase your flexibility and range of motion. Practice the stretches in chapter 6.
■ Add resistance when and where you can.
■ If you can't add resistance, see how slowly you can do some of the exercises.
■ Try multiple sets of some exercises, and see if you get better muscular contractions on the second or

third set. If you don't, go back to one tough set per exercise.

- Every 4 to 6 weeks, change up your routine. Add new exercises you see in the gym, in magazines, or on fitness Web sites. Bring back old favorites. Change your sets and repetitions. Just never do the same ab routine more than 6 weeks in a row without changing something. After 6 weeks, your body will probably have made all the adaptations it's going to make to that routine, and you have to give it something new and challenging to do.
- Give your abs a break every 2 months or so. Take a week off with no abdominal exercise, then start back in with new exercises.

## AEROBICS

You probably don't want to go below the level of cardiovascular exercise you're doing now—1½ hours a week, including 60 minutes in your target heart-rate zone. In fact, if you want to lose weight, you may decide to do significantly more. To keep making improvements in your aerobic fitness and burn off a few more calories, try five aerobic workouts a week. But give yourself variety. Here's what a week's schedule might look like for a jogger.

**Sunday:** A 4- to 5-mile walk-jog
**Monday:** A 30-minute jog
**Tuesday:** Off
**Wednesday:** A hard 2-mile run
**Thursday:** Off
**Friday:** A 30-minute jog

**Saturday:** At least 45 minutes of a completely different aerobic activity (a long bike ride, a canoe trip, a session on an elliptical machine at the gym—anything to put your heart to work while giving your ankles, knees, and lower back a break)

To lose fat while gaining muscle, try interval workouts: After a 5-minute warm-up, go hard for 30 seconds, then easy for 1 minute. Repeat for a total of 10 to 15 minutes. Cool down with 5 easy minutes. This easy-hard combination creates an afterburn effect in which your metabolism remains elevated after the workout, helping you burn more calories. Normal aerobic workouts don't have this effect.

## EATING

The Core Program gave you only a hint of the many ways you can alter your diet to attain a lighter, leaner, more energetic physique. Here are a few more.

**Don't drastically cut the fat in your diet.** That lowers your testosterone, making it harder to build muscle.

**Don't assume that more protein means more muscle.** The protein guidelines in the Core Program aren't minimums; they're the highest levels that have been shown to help build muscle in male weight lifters. Anything beyond that is overkill. Too much protein not only is wasteful but might actually lower your testosterone.

**Avoid all dietary fads.** Almost every big trend that comes along is based on unbalancing your diet: taking away entire macronutrients like carbohydrates or fats, replacing most of your protein with soy, or doing something else that's unnatural, inconvenient, and unsettling. Do you know anyone who's ever made such radical changes and stuck with them for life? Probably not.

Now that you know what you shouldn't do, here's some advice on the dietary habits you should adopt.

**Eat the most of the best.** Try to build most of your meals around the healthiest foods. Many of these are listed in Level One of the Core Program.

**When you indulge, make it short and sweet.** If you crave a particular food, eat it, enjoy it, and get the craving out of your system. The longer you let a craving gnaw at you, the more likely you are to go wild when you finally give in to it.

## THE INEVITABLE SETBACKS

Everyone blows it at one time or another. You get sick and miss a week of training. Or you binge for a few days on a high-stress business trip. Or you get hurt, become depressed because you can't exercise, and sit on the couch and eat all the wrong things. Or you just get bored with what you're doing and fall out of the exercise habit.

What to do? Get back into it slowly, and find a new reason to get excited about what you're doing—a new program or a return to some favorite exercises or a new challenge like training for a 10-K race.

Here are some things to keep in mind when you fall off the washboard wagon.

**You're only a beginner once.** Although your fitness levels fall when you take a layoff, your body has memories of what you were once capable of accomplishing, so you'll return to your previous fitness level faster than you originally attained it.

**You learn from your mistakes.** Think hard about why you had the setback. Did you get sick because you were exercising too hard without a break? Did you get hurt because you did an exercise with bad form? Did you get bored because you went too long without making changes to your routine and stopped seeing results? Your body is a never-ending mystery; there's always a new clue to be discovered that will help you exercise more effectively.

# CHAPTER THIRTEEN

# ESSENTIAL ADVANCED ROUTINES

The nine ab exercises in the Core Program are more than most guys know. But they're not all you need to know. After all, in the previous chapter, we told you to make changes in your exercise routine every 6 weeks. So here are six ways to do things differently.

1. A one-exercise minimalist routine to hit all your abdominal muscles at once
2. An advanced three-exercise routine using equipment you'll find in any gym or health club
3. Seven exercises using a Swiss ball
4. A three-exercise routine for improving sports performance
5. Five very challenging new exercises, any of which you can add to your core ab routine for additional variety
6. A system of circuit routines using exercises you learned in the Core Program

## THE ONE-EXERCISE WONDER

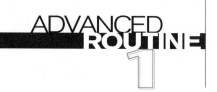

Do 20 repetitions of this exercise to work your upper abs, lower abs, and obliques in one motion. It'll be over with in a minute, so make the most of it: Really focus on feeling your abs work, and strive for perfect technique.

# Double Crunch with a Cross

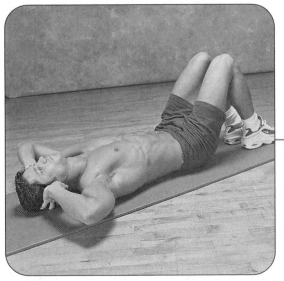

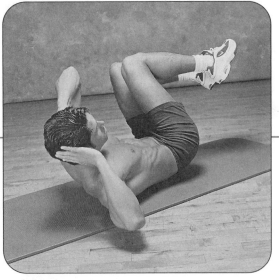

### READY, SET:

Lie on your back with your knees bent, your feet flat on the floor, your head and neck relaxed, and your hands behind your ears.

### GO:

Use your lower abs to lift both knees and cross them toward your left shoulder as you simultaneously use your upper abs to raise your left shoulder and cross it toward your right knee. Hold for a second.

Then, in a controlled motion, slowly lower your legs and torso back to the starting position. As soon as your feet and left shoulder blade lightly touch the floor, do the movement to the other side, raising your knees toward your right shoulder and your right shoulder toward your left knee. That's one repetition.

## PERFORMANCE TIPS

■ Try to raise your hips slightly off the floor on each repetition, as you would in a reverse crunch. It's very hard to do while you're lifting your shoulder blades, but you'll get the best results when you master this double effort.

■ Whether you can get your hips off the floor or not, definitely get your shoulder blades up. Don't just move your neck and head.

# THE GYM ROUTINE

**H**ere are three resistance exercises that require gym equipment, if not a trip to an actual health club. For the hanging knee raise, you need a chin-up bar; you use a dumbbell for the weighted side bend. You might have that gear at home, but you probably don't own the cable machine needed for the cable crunch.

The weights that you use in the weighted side bend and the cable crunch increase the intensity of your workout while keeping your time commitment down. Using weights is an advanced technique, so don't try it until you've progressed through all the levels of the Core Program.

Start with one set of 8 to 12 repetitions of each exercise to get a feel for the movements and the amount of weight you need on the cable crunch and weighted side bend. Do two sets the next week and three the week after. Continue with it as long as you can still increase your repetitions of the hanging knee raise and the amount of weight you use on the cable crunch.

Altogether, you should get a good 5 to 6 weeks—plus some incredible ab development—out of this routine.

# Hanging Knee Raise

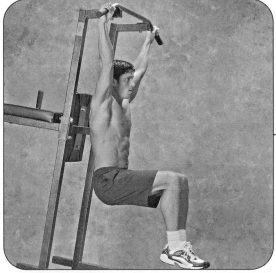

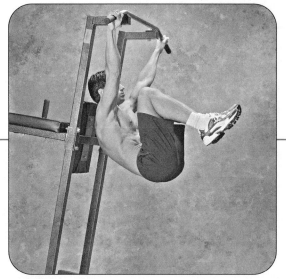

### READY, SET:

Hang from a bar with your hands, or use elbow supports like AbOrigionals (found in many gyms). Or use a Roman chair, supporting yourself with your elbows.

### GO:

Use your lower abs to raise your knees toward your shoulders, curling your pelvis toward your rib cage. Hold for a second.

Then, in a controlled motion, slowly lower yourself back to the starting position. Repeat.

## PERFORMANCE TIPS

■ Your hips should move 2 to 4 inches as they curl up. If you just lift your knees up and down, you work only your hip flexors, muscles on the front of your pelvis that don't have a lot of visual appeal.

■ Pause at the top of the movement and really feel the contraction.

■ Keep your leg swing to a minimum, and always wait until your body stops swinging before you begin the next repetition.

■ If your lower abs are extremely strong and you can easily do three sets of 12 repetitions, hold a light dumbbell between your feet.

■ Another variation is the hanging leg raise, in which you keep your legs straight as you raise them.

# Weighted Side Bend

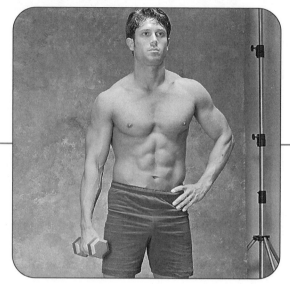 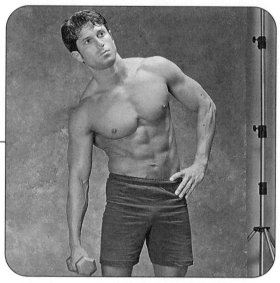

### READY, SET:

Grab a dumbbell in your right hand and let your arm hang straight down from your shoulder. Put your left hand on your left hip, and stand with your feet shoulder-width apart and your knees unlocked.

### GO:

Bend slowly to your right, lowering the dumbbell down your right leg a few inches until you feel a comfortable stretch in your left side.

Then, in a controlled motion, use your left oblique muscles to slowly straighten your body back to the starting position. Repeat. When you finish all of your repetitions on that side, hold the weight in your left hand and do the same number of reps on your other side.

## PERFORMANCE TIPS

■ This is one exercise where you don't want to progressively increase the weight you use. You might start with 10-pound dumbbells, go up to 15s, then maybe go up to 20s and stop there. Why? Because you don't want your oblique muscles to get big and blocky. Some muscle on your sides will look good, contributing to a tapered, athletic look, but if you keep building them, your obliques can overwhelm the rest of your torso.

■ Don't let your torso sway backward or forward; bend straight over your leg.

# Cable Crunch

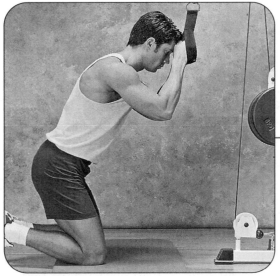
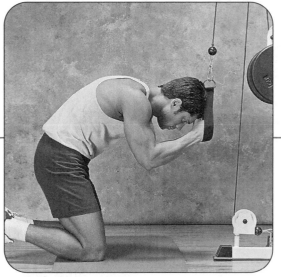

### READY, SET:

Attach a handle to a high cable on a cable machine. Select a light weight. Grab the handle, and kneel facing the machine. Hold the handle in front of your forehead.

### GO:

Without moving your thighs, use your upper abs to curl your torso forward and down. Hold for a second.

Then, in a controlled motion, slowly raise your torso back to the starting position. Repeat.

## PERFORMANCE TIPS

■ This exercise is probably the most effective muscle builder for your upper abs— it'll bring out the six-pack like nothing else. However, it won't work if you don't get the form right. The key is to keep your thighs and hips motionless while you initiate the movement with your upper abs and use them to pull your torso forward and down.

■ You should feel a very intense contraction at the bottom of the movement, almost like a sharp object poking into your ab muscles. That's good; it means you have the right form. Hold that contraction for a second before you release.

## ADVANCED ROUTINE 3

# SWISS MIX

If you belong to a gym, you've probably seen big rubber balls off in the corner. Maybe you've seen a trainer using one with a client or a few gym members doing abdominal exercises on them.

They go by a number of names: Swiss balls, thera-balls, resista-balls. No matter what you call them, they offer a big benefit to someone looking for better abdominal muscles. They allow you to start each repetition from a pre-stretch position. That is, instead of starting a crunch from a flat position on the floor, you start with your back arched. That means a longer range of motion, more work for your abdominal muscles, and more benefit from each repetition.

A secondary benefit is that the ball isn't stable. If you don't carefully balance, the ball will move and you'll fall off. So you end up using muscles in your midsection, hips, and thighs to hold your body in place on the ball. It will take a few workouts to get the hang of the exercises, but once you do, you'll quickly realize how much harder your muscles are working, and you'll soon see the results of that extra effort.

The following exercises can be done as a single routine in which you do one to three sets of each exercise. Or you can mix and match, trying any of the Swiss ball exercises with other ab moves that you like. However you do them, try to do 10 to 15 repetitions per set on most of the exercises. On the Swiss ball reverse crunch, 6 to 10 reps are plenty. And on the Swiss ball bridge, try to hold one position for as long as possible, shooting for one to five repetitions of 10 to 30 seconds each.

# Swiss Ball Reverse Crunch

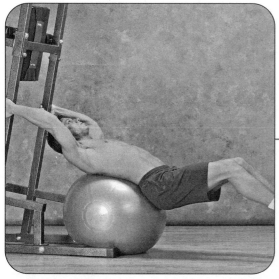

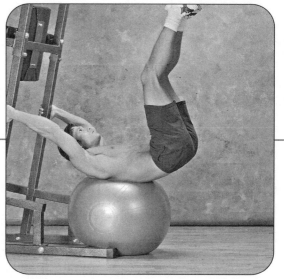

### READY, SET:

Set the ball next to something you can grab on to: a bar, rail, or pole. Lie on your back on the ball, reach behind you, and grip the bar. Your hips should be lower than your shoulders, with your legs extended out in front of you and your knees slightly bent.

### GO:

Use your lower abs to raise your legs and crunch your pelvis toward your rib cage. Hold for a second.

Then, in a controlled motion, slowly lower your legs back to the starting position. Repeat.

## PERFORMANCE TIPS

■ Throughout the movement, keep your back arched around the ball and your head back. Your body's instinct will be to raise your head so you can watch your feet, but you have to remind yourself to keep your head in the same position throughout the exercise. This reduces strain on your neck.

■ As in all lower-ab exercises, the key is rotating your pelvis upward. Just raising your legs up and down without also lifting your hips up off the ball means that your hip flexors are doing most of the work.

# Swiss Ball Jackknife

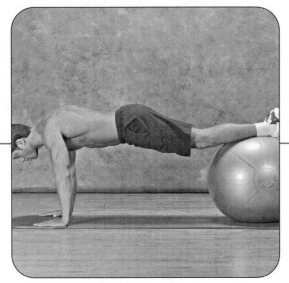 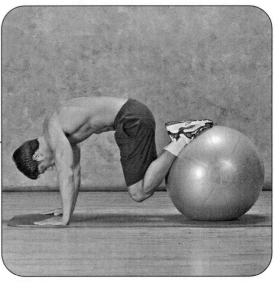

### READY, SET:

Rest your hands on the floor and the fronts of your lower legs on the ball, as if you were going to do a pushup.

### GO:

Use your lower abs to pull your knees as far forward as possible. Hold for a second.

Then, in a controlled motion, slowly straighten your legs back to the starting position. Repeat.

## PERFORMANCE TIPS

- Start the exercise with your back flat—neither rounded upward nor arched downward. This means your abs will be slightly contracted before you start the exercise.

- At the end of the movement, your back should still be flat or, even better, rounded upward; this means your abdominal muscles are fully contracted.

- Keep your head down in the pushup position throughout the exercise. It's okay to let your head drop farther toward the floor, but you'll defeat the purpose of the exercise if you raise your head.

# Swiss Ball Side-Lying Oblique Crunch

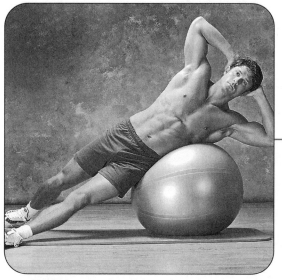 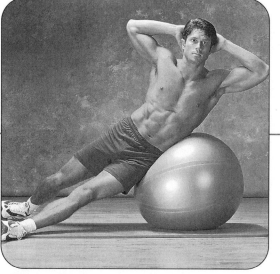

### READY, SET:

Lie on your left side on the ball, with your legs in a scissor position on the floor: left foot forward, right foot back. Keep your head and neck relaxed, with your hands behind your ears or head.

### GO:

Use your right obliques to raise the right side of your rib cage toward the right side of your pelvis. Hold for a second.

Then, in a controlled motion, slowly lower yourself back to the starting position. Repeat.

When you finish all of your repetitions on your right side, switch positions to work your left side: Lie on your right side and do the same number of reps on your left side.

## PERFORMANCE TIPS

■ Start the movement with your oblique muscles rather than your head and shoulders. Your head should stay in alignment with your spine throughout the movement, rather than move from side to side.

■ Try to get as high up on the ball as you can while keeping your feet on the floor. The object is to start the exercise with your body almost parallel to the floor. The closer you get to that position, the more your muscles work against gravity, which will give you the best results.

# Swiss Ball Rotational Crunch

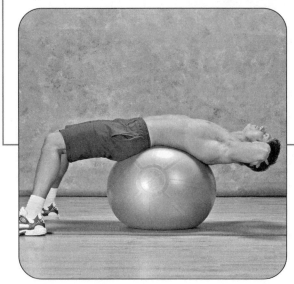 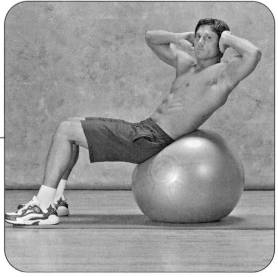

### READY, SET:

Lie on your back on the ball with your feet flat on the floor, your back curved around the ball, and your hands behind your ears or head.

### GO:

Use your upper abs to raise your torso until your upper abs are fully contracted. Continue the movement with a twist to your left.

Return to the starting position and repeat, this time twisting to your right. That's one repetition.

## PERFORMANCE TIPS

■ As in any crunch, keep a fist's distance between your chin and chest.

■ Keep your head aligned with your spine throughout the movement. As you get tired, you'll be tempted to just move your head and elbows in a circle. By keeping your head in a fixed alignment, you force your abdominal muscles to move your entire upper torso.

■ Each workout, switch the side on which you start: If you crunch to the left and then to the right in the first workout, reverse that order and start with a crunch to the right the next time you do Swiss ball rotational crunches.

# Swiss Ball Crunch

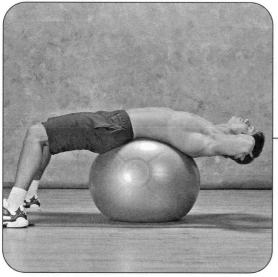 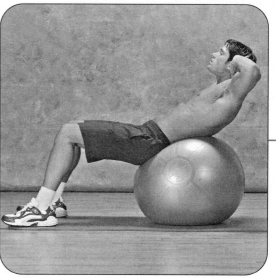

### READY, SET:

Lie on your back on the ball with your feet flat on the floor, your back curved around the ball, and your hands behind your ears or head.

### GO:

Use your upper abs to raise your rib cage toward your pelvis and lift your shoulders up off the ball. Hold for a second.

Then, in a controlled motion, slowly return to the starting position. Repeat.

## PERFORMANCE TIPS

■ Even if regular crunches don't feel challenging to you anymore, the Swiss ball crunch will probably be tough the first time you try it. The ball adds as much as 15 degrees to your range of motion.

■ As you get used to the longer motion and find you can easily do sets of 15 repetitions, add weight by holding a dumbbell under your chin. Remember, though, to keep you head and neck aligned with your torso and to maintain a fist's distance between your chin and chest.

# Swiss Ball Bridge

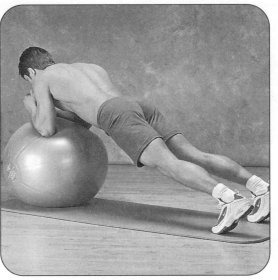

### READY, SET, GO:

Rest your forearms on the ball and your toes on the floor, with your body forming a straight line. Pull your stomach in, trying to bring your belly button back to your spine, and hold, breathing steadily.

## PERFORMANCE TIPS

- At first, you may not be able to hold this for more than 5 to 10 seconds at a time. Do several repetitions of these short holds, trying to build up to one or two repetitions of about 30 seconds.

- By pulling your stomach in and holding it, you're working a muscle called your transverse abdominis. This is a deep strap of muscle that helps hold your internal organs in place. Training it can give your waist a permanently slimmer appearance.

- The Swiss ball bridge builds strength and endurance in your lower back and abdominals simultaneously. If you reverse the position, putting your forearms on the floor and your feet on the ball, you increase the challenge to your lower back.

# Swiss Ball Back Extension

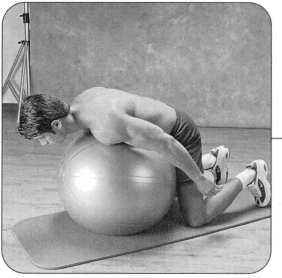 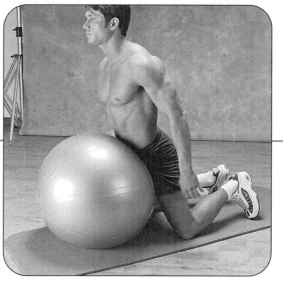

### READY, SET:

Kneel with the ball against the fronts of your thighs and drape the front of your torso over it, with your arms at your sides.

### GO:

Use your lower-back muscles to straighten your torso. Hold for a second.

Then, in a controlled motion, slowly return to the starting position. Repeat.

## PERFORMANCE TIPS

■ Keep your thighs in a fixed position; you want all the movement to occur in your back.

■ If your back is strong and you find this exercise easy, you can hold your hands behind your ears, out in front of you, or out to the sides. That will increase the challenge to your back muscles.

■ For an even bigger challenge, you can hold your hands out to the sides while holding light weights.

# ABS FOR SPORTS

**E**ver hear the expression "He's in great health-club shape, but he's not in game shape"? This describes an athlete who has been training hard in a gym and, to the untrained eye, appears to be in great shape. But he hasn't developed sport-specific speed and power. There's a big difference between the two types of fitness.

Muscle is most efficiently built with slow, controlled movements. But success in sports isn't about having bigger muscles than your opponent (unless the sport is bodybuilding, of course). It's about being able to react to a change in the flow of a game and get to a spot faster than an opponent: Picture a point guard quickly twisting in one direction to steal a pass and then just as quickly changing direction to start a fast break. Or it's about throwing or striking an object as hard as possible: Think of Ken Griffey Jr. whacking a tape measure home run or Tiger Woods turning St. Andrews into a pitch-and-putt course with his intercontinental drives.

So does this mean that the exercises you do in the Core Program are a waste of time if you're interested in sports? No. They build basic strength and endurance in your abdominals. The athletes just mentioned build this foundation with isolated movements before moving on to more advanced movements. Each needs to be able to quickly rotate his torso to achieve his goal. He's not thinking about how he's contracting his abdominals as he does these things. But training his abdominals to move fast and powerfully helps him perform at his expert level.

Once you have built a base of abdominal strength, you need to do exercises more specific to athletic power if you want to use your gym workouts to improve what you do outside the gym. The following three-exercise workout will give you an idea of the difference between training for muscle and training for speed and power. Start cautiously as you learn the exercises, then gradually build up speed.

Begin with one set of 10 to 15 repetitions. Build up to three sets, working in circuit fashion by finishing a set of each exercise before repeating any of them.

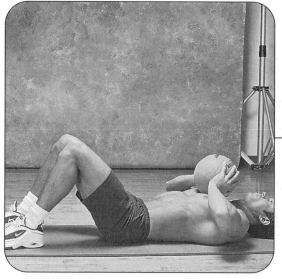

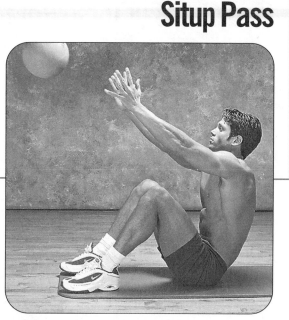

### READY, SET:

Grab a basketball and hold it against your chest. Lie on your back, 4 to 5 feet away from and perpendicular to a wall, with your knees bent and your feet flat on the floor. Keep your head and neck relaxed.

### GO:

Raise your torso quickly, and throw the ball to the wall.

Stay up until the ball comes back to you, catch it, and pull it to your chest. Then, in a controlled motion, slowly lower yourself back to the starting position. As soon as your shoulder blades lightly touch the floor, repeat.

## PERFORMANCE TIPS

■ This is a situp, not a crunch, so you're supposed to use your hip flexor muscles as well as your upper abs. You'll still feel a pretty good contraction in your abs as you hold the situp position and wait for the ball to come back off the wall.

■ As you get used to the exercise, start farther from the wall so you have to throw the ball harder and wait longer to catch it.

■ This move has many variations. You can do it without a ball, making the throwing motion with just your hands. Or you can use a partner, throwing the ball to him and catching it when he throws it back. Finally, if you have a partner, you can use a medicine ball, which will make the exercise much tougher and more beneficial.

# Medicine Ball Torso Rotation

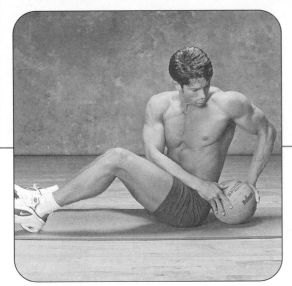 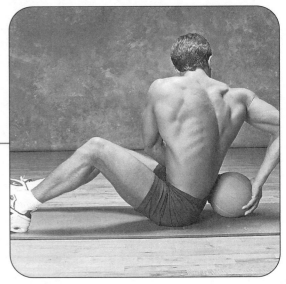

### READY, SET:

Hold a medicine ball or basketball in front of you. Sit with your knees bent and your feet on the floor. Quickly twist to your left and set the ball behind your back.

### GO:

Twist to your right, and pick up the ball.

Bring the ball around to your left, and set it down again. Repeat.

When you finish all of your repetitions in which you twist first to your left side, do the same number of reps in the opposite direction: Twist first to your right to put the ball behind your back, then twist to your left to pick it back up.

## PERFORMANCE TIPS

- You'll quickly realize that you need a lot of torso flexibility to set the ball down directly behind your back and then pick it up again. The stretches in chapter 6 will help you gain that flexibility.

- If you don't have a ball, try the exercise with a light dumbbell. Grab the weights on the ends of the dumbbell, not the bar in the middle.

# Woodchopper

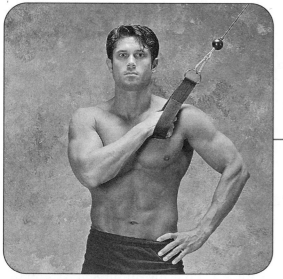  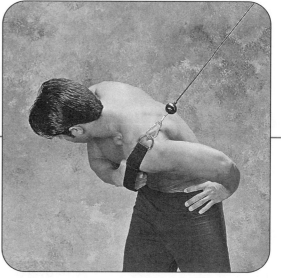

## READY, SET:

Attach a handle to a high cable on a cable machine. Select a light weight. Grab the handle with your right hand, and stand with the left side of your body facing the weight stack. Hold the handle up near your left shoulder.

## GO:

Moving only at your waist, bend to your right, pulling the handle down toward your right hip. Hold for a second.

Then, in a controlled motion, slowly return to the starting position. Repeat.

When you finish all of your repetitions on that side, switch positions to work your other side: Stand with your right side facing the weights, grasp the handle with your left hand, and bend to your left. Do the same number of reps on that side.

## PERFORMANCE TIPS

■ Your shoulders will rotate a little, but you want to make sure that you initiate the movement with your obliques.

■ Keep your hips facing forward throughout the movement. If they move, they take work away from your obliques.

ADVANCED
ROUTINE
5

# CHALLENGING CHANGE-UP

**H**ere are three tough exercises to test your middle's mettle after you have mastered the Core Program. We don't necessarily mean for you to treat these as their own ab routine—feel free to mix and match them with the Core Program exercises to avoid boredom.

The recommended number of reps varies depending upon the difficulty of the exercise. Refer to the "Performance Tips" for each exercise to see the number of reps you should shoot for.

When doing the weighted crunch and weighted reverse crunch, start out by using just 5 pounds. This may not seem like much, but if you maintain proper technique and isolate your abs, you will feel the difference.

If you progress to the point of using heavy weights (25 pounds or more), you may start to gain more mass on your abs than you want. So keep an eye on things. You can overtrain any muscle, creating an imbalance and destroying your body's natural symmetry.

# Bent-Knee Leg Over

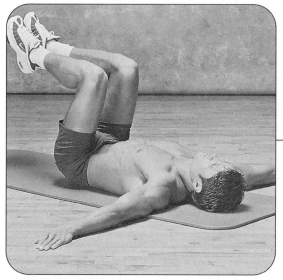

## READY, SET:

Lie on your back with your hands palms-down and spread straight out, perpendicular to your body. Keep your head and neck relaxed. You want your lower body to form two right angles: Your thighs should be perpendicular to your upper body, with your lower legs parallel to the floor.

## GO:

Slowly lower your legs to your left side until your left leg lightly touches the floor. Hold for a second.

Then, in a controlled motion, use your right obliques to slowly raise your legs back to the starting position. As soon as your legs reach the upright position, do the movement to your other side. That's one repetition.

## PERFORMANCE TIPS

- Do 12 repetitions in your first workout, 13 in your second, and 14 in your third. The next week, start with 16 reps and work up to 18.

- Allow your hips to roll along with your legs.

- Keep your shoulders flat on the floor.

- Use your obliques to slow the descent of your legs to the side. This negative portion of the repetition is just as important as the positive phase for building strength and endurance in your oblique muscles.

- Don't rest the weight of your legs on the floor during the pause on each side.

- Roll your head from side to side with your legs or keep it in one place.

# Weighted Crunch

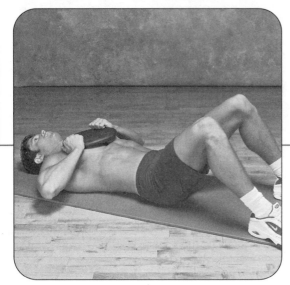 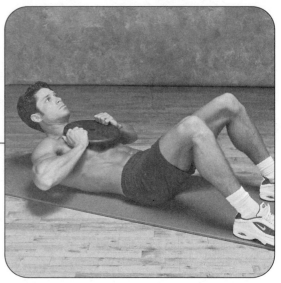

### READY, SET:

Lie on your back holding a weight plate or dumbbell at chin level, with your knees bent and your feet flat on the floor. Keep your head and neck relaxed.

### GO:

Use your upper abs to raise your rib cage toward your pelvis and lift your shoulder blades off the floor. Hold for a second.

Then, in a controlled motion, slowly lower your shoulders back to the starting position. As soon as your shoulder blades lightly touch the floor, repeat.

## PERFORMANCE TIPS

- Start with 10 repetitions and work up to 12. When you can easily do 12, increase the weight and decrease the reps back to 10, then work back up to 12.

- As with any crunch, make sure you keep a fist's distance between your chin and chest.

- The first few times you do weighted crunches, you may be surprised at how quickly your body poops out on you. Don't worry about getting all the recommended repetitions if you can't do them with good form. Just nodding your head up off the floor won't help you build your abdominals.

# Weighted Reverse Crunch

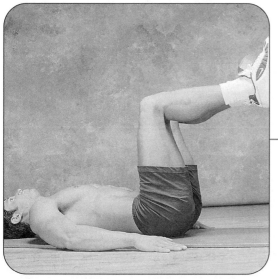
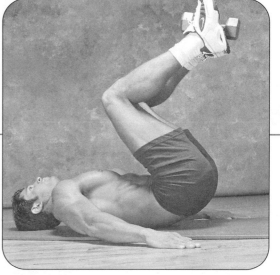

### READY, SET:

Lie on your back with your head and neck relaxed and a dumbbell between your feet. You want your lower body to form two right angles: Your thighs should be perpendicular to your upper body, with your lower legs parallel to the floor.

### GO:

Use your lower abs to raise your hips off the floor and toward your rib cage. Hold for a second.

Then, in a controlled motion, slowly lower your hips back to the starting position. As they lightly touch the floor, repeat.

## PERFORMANCE TIPS

- Start with 10 repetitions and work up to 12. When you can easily do 12, increase the weight and decrease the reps back to 10, then work back up to 12.

- Make sure your lower abs do the work. If you just lift your legs up and down without getting your hips up off the floor and tilting your pelvis toward your rib cage, you're not working your ab muscles.

- Don't rest your hips on the floor at the bottom of the movement or let your lower legs drop down.

- Keep constant tension on your abs.

- Use your hands for stability, not to press your hips upward.

- You can also hold a medicine ball between your feet or knees on this exercise.

# CIRCUIT CITY

In the Core Program, you tried to do a suggested number of repetitions of each exercise. Now, you're going to try to do some of those exercises for a specific length of time. The actual number of repetitions you do will vary according to how fast you do them.

In circuit training, you move quickly from one exercise to the next without resting. This increases your heart rate, adding an aerobic aspect to your workout. The circuits are divided into rounds. A round is complete when you have performed each of the exercises in the circuit for the specified length of time. Your goal is to work up to five rounds of circuits one and two and two rounds of circuit three, resting for 5 seconds between rounds. Until you build up endurance, you may need to rest for up to 30 seconds. But the object is to give your abs a nearly continuous workout for 5 minutes. Go at your own pace, and stop when you have a breakdown in technique.

You can do the circuits as a progressive program, much like the Core Program. Do each circuit for 2 weeks, then move on to the next. Or, for a change of pace, you can do any one of the circuits at random without worrying about progression—it'll give your muscles an interesting new challenge.

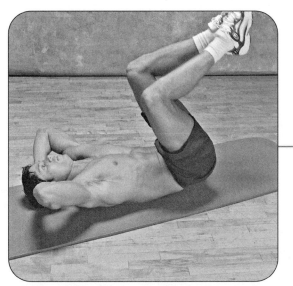
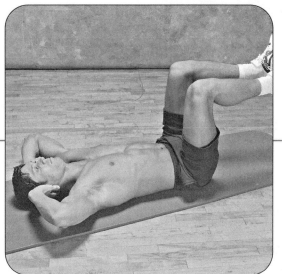

**REVERSE CRUNCH:** Raise and lower your hips for 30 seconds (15 to 20 repetitions).

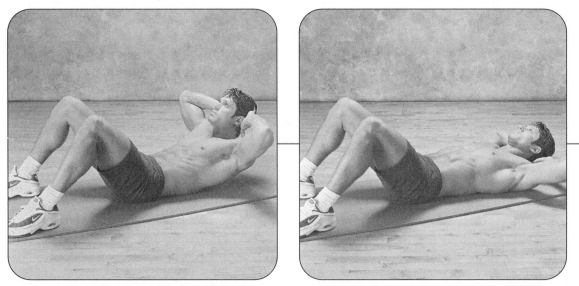

**CRUNCH: FEET FLAT:** Raise your rib cage and lift your shoulder blades, then lower. Repeat for 30 seconds (15 to 20 repetitions).

▲ *If you need a refresher on the specific instructions for these exercises, see pages 54 and 56.*

# With a Twist

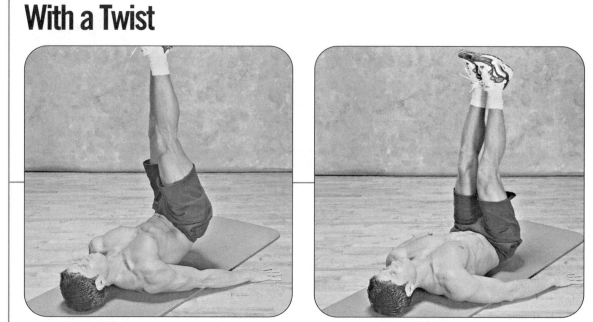

**CORKSCREW:** Raise and twist your hips and legs, lower, then raise and twist to the other side. Repeat for 30 seconds (7 to 10 repetitions to each side).

▲ *If you need a refresher on the specific instructions for this exercise, see page 77.*

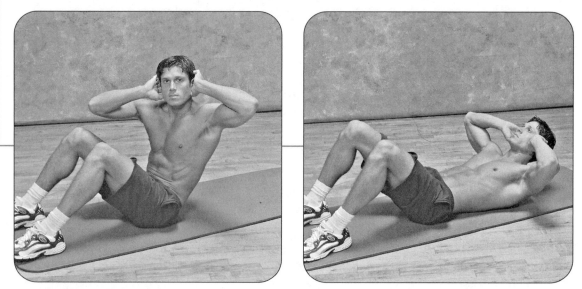

**CRUNCH WITH A CROSS:** Raise your rib cage, lift your shoulder blades, cross one shoulder toward the opposite knee, lower, then raise and cross to the other side. Repeat for 30 seconds (7 to 10 repetitions to each side).

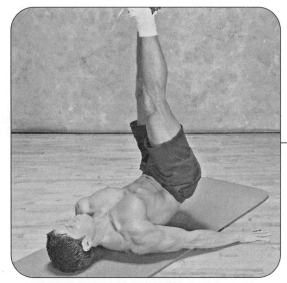

CORKSCREW: Raise and twist your hips and legs, lower, then raise and twist to the other side. Repeat for 30 seconds (7 to 10 repetitions to each side).

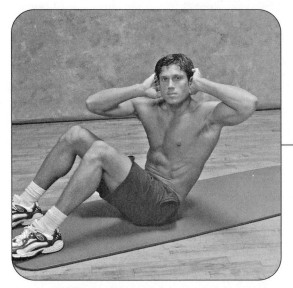

CRUNCH WITH A CROSS: Raise your rib cage, lift your shoulder blades, cross one shoulder toward the opposite knee, lower, then raise and cross to the other side. Repeat for 30 seconds (7 to 10 repetitions to each side).

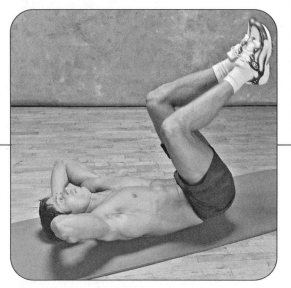

REVERSE CRUNCH: Raise and lower your hips for 30 seconds (15 to 20 repetitions).

*(continued)*

# Five Alive (cont.)

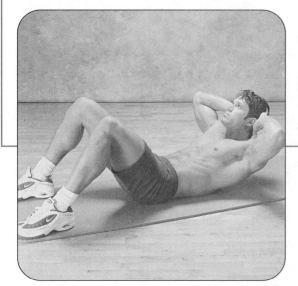

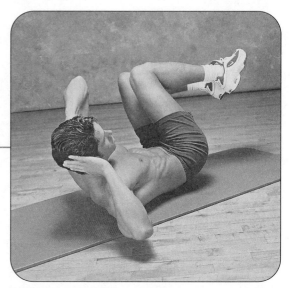

**CRUNCH: FEET FLAT:** Raise your rib cage and lift your shoulder blades, then lower. Repeat for 30 seconds (15 to 20 repetitions).

**DOUBLE CRUNCH WITH A CROSS:** Simultaneously raise your knees and one shoulder and cross them toward each other, lower, then raise and cross to the other side. Repeat for 30 seconds (7 to 10 repetitions to each side).

▲ *If you need a refresher on the specific instructions for these exercises, see pages 77, 122, 79, 69, and 99.*

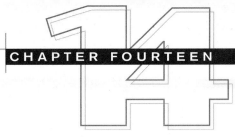

# CHAPTER FOURTEEN

# ESSENTIAL
# WEIGHTS
## STRENGTH TRAINING

Now that you know what it feels like to have a tighter, stronger midsection, you probably wonder what it would be like to have an entire body like that.

The only way to find out is to start doing total-body strength training three times a week. When you pump iron—or do any resistance exercise, whether it's a crunch, pushup, pullup, dip, or bench press—you force your body to make important adaptations. It quickly gets stronger as it sorts out the new stimuli and starts recruiting more and more muscle fibers and nerve cells to help with the task of lifting these heavy things. After 4 to 8 weeks, it runs out of fresh muscles and nerves and must do something truly radical: Make the muscle cells larger.

If this information sounds vaguely familiar, it's because this is exactly the process you've gone through with your abdominal muscles. This chapter will tell you how to start it over again with the muscles in your chest, back, shoulders, arms, butt, and legs.

Besides pumping up those muscles, total-body strength training also reinforces your well-defined abs by increasing your muscle mass, which in turn cranks up your metabolism, the speed with which your body burns calories all day. Adding a pound of muscle increases your metabolic rate by as much as 50 calories a day. Five extra pounds of muscle could burn an additional 250 calories a day, or 1,750 a week.

## BENEFITS OF STRENGTH TRAINING

**Strengthens your entire body**

**Builds bone mass**

**Speeds up your metabolism, or the number of calories your body burns on a minute-by-minute basis, leading to less body fat**

**Lowers your blood pressure**

**Decreases cortisol, a stress hormone that signals your body to store abdominal fat**

**Helps your body hold on to its fast-twitch muscle fibers, which rapidly diminish with age; if they're not used in strength-building activities, they're permanently lost**

Way back in chapter 2, you learned that a pound of fat contains 3,500 calories. With 5 more pounds of muscle on your body, you'd burn an extra pound of fat every 2 weeks.

Now, where are you going to build 5 pounds of muscle? Certainly not in your midsection alone. Abdominal muscles are pretty small, so when you build your abs, it has only a limited effect on your metabolism.

But a whole-body strength-training program can put muscle on your chest, back, shoulders, and legs. It will not only look good there, giving your body a younger, stronger, more athletic appearance, but also help you burn more calories, 24 hours a day, 7 days a week.

Strength training your larger muscles also creates surges in your production of testosterone and growth hormone. Training smaller muscles, like your abs, won't help your body generate these powerful muscle-building, fat-burning hormones.

## THE BASIC-EIGHT ROUTINE

The Basic Eight is a simple workout requiring just dumbbells and a bench. You can do it at home or in a gym. Here are a few specifics.

■ If you want to do these exercises on the same day as your Core Program workout, use this order: abdominal exercises, Basic Eight, aerobics. If you do aerobics before strength training, you'll exhaust your body's energy stores before you lift, diminishing the benefits of the strength program. If you do your strength training on one of your ab rest days, warm up for 5 minutes before beginning.

■ Do the exercises in the order in which they're listed. As a general rule, you should always work bigger muscles (back, chest, gluteals, thighs) before smaller muscles (arms, calves).

■ There's no rule about how much weight to start with. In general, it's better to start with something a little lighter than what you think you can lift. If it's too light and you can do all the repetitions easily, just increase the weight the next time you lift. And it's not the end of the world if you pick a starting weight that's too ambitious and can't do enough repetitions; just try something lighter the next time, and build up from there.

■ Do one set of each of the eight exercises, resting as little as possible between exercises.

■ Do 10 to 15 repetitions of each upper-body exercise. (For the arm exercises, that means 10 to 15 with each arm.) When you can do 15 repetitions with a particular weight, increase to a weight that's challenging for 10 repetitions.

■ Do 15 to 20 repetitions of lower-body exercises. (That's 15 to 20 with each leg on the lunges.) When you can do 20 reps with a weight, increase to a weight that's challenging for 15 reps.

# Squat (Thighs and Gluteals)

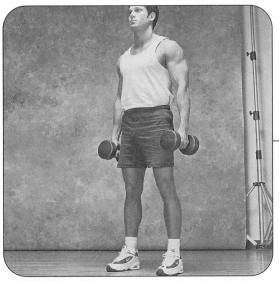

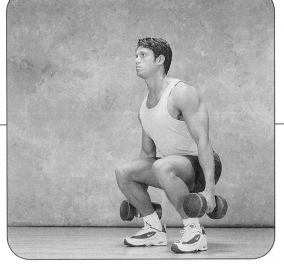

## READY, SET:

Hold a pair of dumbbells and let your arms hang straight down from your shoulders. Stand with your feet a little wider than shoulder-width apart, your toes pointed slightly out, and your knees slightly bent. Pull your shoulders back, push your chest out, and look straight ahead. Your lower back should be neither arched nor rounded, and your head should be in alignment with your spine.

## GO:

Bend your knees to lower yourself, and as you sink, sit back as if you were heading for a chair. Go down slowly until your thighs are parallel to the floor or until your heels start to rise off the floor.

Slowly rise back up to the starting position, and repeat.

## PERFORMANCE TIPS

- ■ Try this without weights at first. Hold your hands straight out from your shoulders.

- ■ On the squat, flexibility and strength are intertwined. Keep your heels flat on the floor and your back in its natural alignment. You'll get the most benefit when you can descend until your upper thighs are parallel to the floor. It may take weeks or months to put these components together, but when you do, you'll develop muscle fast.

- ■ Squats will make your knee joints stronger as long as you do them in a controlled fashion. Never lower yourself rapidly or bounce out of the bottom position—that is too tough on your knees and doesn't do your lower back any favors.

# Lunge (Thighs and Gluteals)

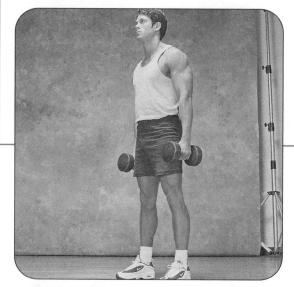
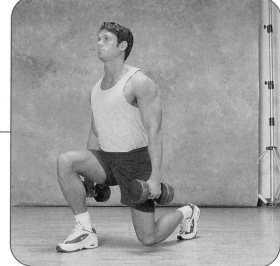

### READY, SET:

Hold a pair of dumbbells and let your arms hang straight down from your shoulders. Stand with your feet a little wider than shoulder-width apart, your toes pointed slightly out, and your knees slightly bent. Pull your shoulders back, push your chest out, and look straight ahead. Your lower back should be neither arched nor rounded, and your head should be in alignment with your spine.

### GO:

With your nondominant leg, step a little farther forward than you would in a normal stride, and land on your heel as you bend that knee 90 degrees and lower your other knee until it's just short of touching the floor.

Push back off your forward heel and return to the starting position. You can either finish all your reps with the same leg forward before switching to the other leg or alternate legs until you finish the set.

## PERFORMANCE TIPS

- Try this without weights at first. When you can do 20 reps with each leg, add the dumbbells.

- Start with your weaker leg, and always do the same number of repetitions with each leg. If you start with your stronger side, you may not be able to finish the same number with your weaker one, increasing your strength discrepancy.

- Lengthen your stride until you can bend your forward knee 90 degrees and still keep it behind your toes. Never bounce your back knee off the ground.

- Keep your torso upright throughout the set. It'll drift forward as you get tired, but keeping it straight forces your lower back and abs to do more work.

# Bench Press (Chest, Triceps, and Shoulders)

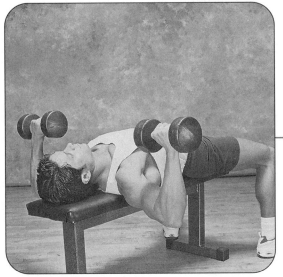 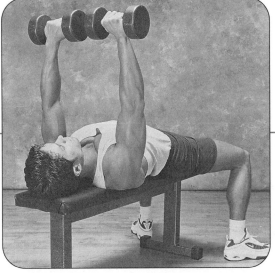

**READY, SET:**

Grab a pair of dumbbells in an overhand grip. Lie on a bench with your feet flat on the floor for stability. Hold the weights just above and outside your chest.

**GO:**

Push the weights up in a slanting motion so they almost meet when your arms are fully extended.

Slowly lower to the starting position, pause, and repeat.

## PERFORMANCE TIPS

- Most guys who haven't lifted before have a strength discrepancy, meaning that one arm is stronger than the other, especially if they play sports that use one arm more than the other. So it may be tough at first to get both dumbbells moving at the same speed and in the same range of motion. Once you get the coordination down, your strength will increase rapidly—and equally.

- Keep your lower back in its natural position throughout the exercise. Don't allow it to arch excessively so you can push up heavier weights.

- Don't clank the weights together at the top. It takes tension off your muscles.

- Lower the weights as far as they want to go—that's your natural range of motion on this exercise. If you try to stop them short of a full descent or lower them past your comfort zone, you risk straining your shoulders and limiting your gains.

- A pushup works the same muscles as a bench press, so if you want extra work for your chest, add a set of pushups right after your presses. Do as many as you can.

# Bent-Over Row (Upper Back and Biceps)

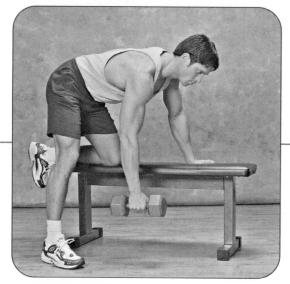 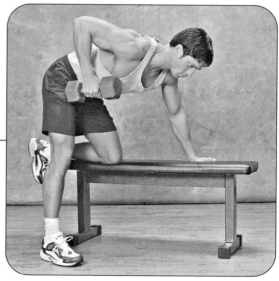

**READY, SET:**

Hold a dumbbell with your nondominant hand, palm facing in, and let your arm hang straight down from your shoulder. Put your opposite hand and knee on a bench so that your upper body is at slightly more than a 90-degree angle. Tighten your abs for stability.

**GO:**

Pull the weight straight up toward the side of your abdomen.

Pause, then slowly lower the weight back to the starting position. Pause again, and repeat.

When you finish all your repetitions on your nondominant side, switch positions to work your dominant side: Hold the dumbbell in your dominant hand and do the same number of reps on that side.

## PERFORMANCE TIPS

■ Start with your weaker arm, and do the same number of reps with each side.

■ Focus on your back muscles: Concentrate on their pulling your arm back to start the movement, rather than on starting the movement with your arm.

■ Keep your torso in one fixed position throughout the exercise. If you add any body rotation to the movement, you take your back muscles out of the exercise.

■ Pause at the top and bottom of the movement, and lower the weight slowly to work your back muscles on the way up and the way down.

# Calf Raise

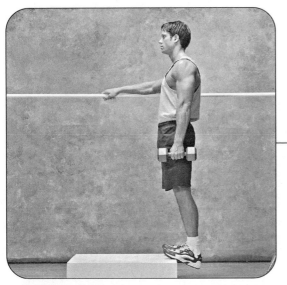
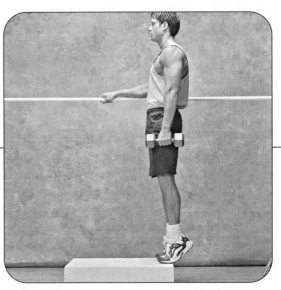

### READY, SET:

Hold a dumbbell and let your arm hang straight down from your shoulder. Stand on the balls of your feet on a raised step or platform (a staircase works well) with your feet hip-width apart and your heels hanging off the platform, as low as they'll go. Use your free hand to hold on to whatever you can for support.

### GO:

Raise your heels as high as possible, distributing your weight toward your big toes.

Pause, then slowly return to the starting position. Pause again, and repeat.

## PERFORMANCE TIPS

- Each workout, alternate the hand in which you hold the weight. Or do half the repetitions with the weight in one hand, then switch for the other half.

- You may prefer to work one calf at a time. Tuck the nonworking foot behind your working calf, and hold the weight on the side you're working.

- Don't turn your toes in and out to try to work different sides of your calves. That's not how the muscles work.

- Always go as high as you can and as low as you can on each repetition, and pause for a full second in each position. You'll build the most muscle this way.

# Rotation Press (Shoulders and Triceps)

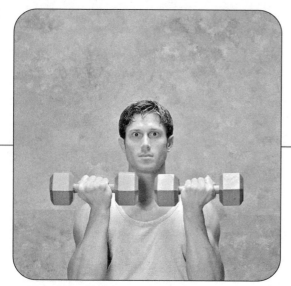 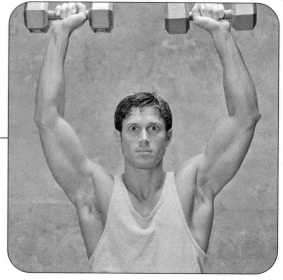

### READY, SET:

Grab a pair of dumbbells and stand with your feet shoulder-width apart and your knees slightly bent. Hold the weights at chin level with your hands rotated so the backs face forward. Pull your shoulders back, push your chest out, and look straight ahead.

### GO:

Push the weights up directly over your head, rotating your hands so your palms face forward when your arms are fully extended.

Pause, then slowly lower the weights to the starting position, rotating your hands back again, and repeat.

## PERFORMANCE TIPS

■ Keep your legs and torso in the same position throughout the lift. Don't allow yourself to lean back as you push the weights over your head—that's murder on your lower back.

■ Don't bring the dumbbells together at the top; your shoulders will work harder if you keep the weights apart.

■ Watch your knees. It's tempting to bend them a little as you lower the weight and then straighten them as you lift again. But that's a different exercise, called a push press, which is good for sports training but not the ideal way to build shoulder muscles. You want to do all the work with your shoulders, not split it up with bigger, lower-body muscles.

# Biceps Curl

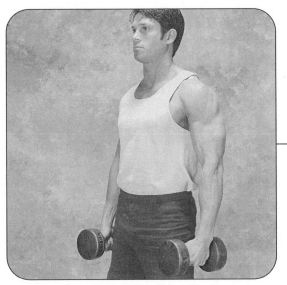
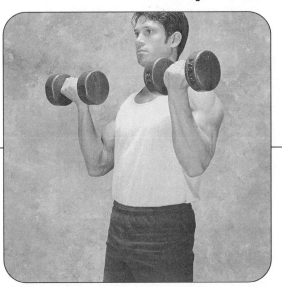

## READY, SET:

Hold a pair of dumbbells and let your arms hang straight down from your shoulders. Keep your upper arms tight against your sides. Stand with your feet shoulder-width apart.

## GO:

Bend at your elbows to begin the curl, and as the weights curl upward, rotate your palms until they're facing straight up. Stop the movement when you can't lift the weights any farther without moving your upper arms.

Pause, then slowly lower the weights to the starting position, rotating your hands back again. Pause again, and repeat.

## PERFORMANCE TIPS

■ Keep your upper arms motionless and pressed against your upper torso throughout the range of movement. If you move them, you incorporate shoulder muscles into the exercise.

■ Control the dumbbells on the way down. You'll develop more muscle in your arms with a slower lowering.

■ To make the exercise harder and build muscle faster, try standing with your back flat against a wall for support. You'll be amazed at how much harder the exercise is when your back is immobilized like this.

# Kickback (Triceps)

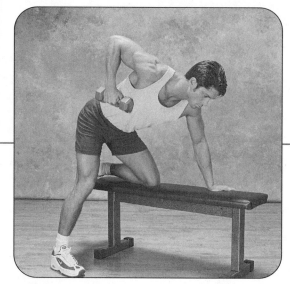

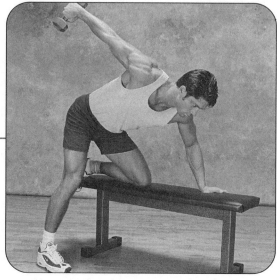

**READY, SET:**

Hold a dumbbell with your nondominant hand, palm facing in. Put your opposite hand and knee on a bench so that your upper body is at slightly more than a 90-degree angle. Raise the dumbbell to the side of your abdomen, and point your elbow up toward the ceiling.

**GO:**

Keeping your elbow pointing straight up, straighten your arm.

Pause, feel the squeeze in your triceps, then slowly lower the weight back to the starting position. Repeat. When you finish all of your repetitions with your nondominant side, switch positions: Hold the dumbbell in your dominant hand and do the same number of reps on that side.

## PERFORMANCE TIPS

■ Start with your weaker arm, and do the same number of reps with each side.

■ Most people do this exercise with their upper arms parallel to the floor. If you do that, your triceps have to work in only the last couple of inches of your range of motion; there's no resistance from gravity until you get to that point. Keep your upper arm perpendicular to the floor so you fight gravity all the way up.

■ Keep your torso fixed in one place. If you move it, you add momentum to the exercise, taking work away from your triceps.

## MOVING ON UP

You can do the Basic Eight for 6 to 8 weeks, with the following modifications.

■ After 2 weeks, increase to two sets of each exercise. But drop the repetitions. Do 10 to 12 repetitions of the upper-body exercises and 12 to 15 reps of the lower-body exercises.

■ After 4 weeks, increase to three sets, but drop the repetitions further: 8 to 10 for your upper body, 10 to 12 for your lower body.

■ Finally, spend 2 weeks using a pyramid system: Start each exercise with a set of 10 to 12 repetitions, then do a heavier set of 8 to 10, then an even heavier set of 6 to 8.

After 6 weeks, take a week off, then come back with a new program consisting of new exercises and new numbers of sets and reps.

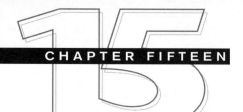

# CHAPTER FIFTEEN

# ESSENTIAL LONG-RANGE PLAN

The longer you train, the more you learn about your body's strengths and weaknesses. You'll try lots of different programs, lots of combinations of your favorite exercises and interesting new ones.

But no matter what you do, your body will always undergo changes in a set pattern. Let's take a closer look at this pattern, which is called the general adaptation syndrome (remember this in case you ever feel like impressing your fellow gym rats while you're standing around the drinking fountain). The general adaptation syndrome, developed during the 1930s, shows that there are three stages to the training process: the alarm stage, the resistance stage, and the exhaustion, or overwork, stage.

## #1
## ALARM STAGE

This is your body's initial response to exercise. During this stage, you are liable to get mildly sore, really sore, or hurt. Your goal when starting a new exercise program is to minimize the negative effects of the alarm stage. If you give your body too big a shock in the beginning, there's a good chance that you'll quit the program before you've had a chance to get to the next stage.

## #2
## RESISTANCE STAGE

At this point, you start to see the benefits of the new program. You'll experience three types of improvements: physiological (your muscles respond by getting bigger and stronger), mechanical (you get better at the exercises), and psychological (getting bigger, stronger, and better bolsters your self-confidence and prompts you to push yourself harder and bump up the intensity of your workouts).

But if you push yourself too hard, you find yourself in the third stage.

## #3
## EXHAUSTION, OR OVERWORK, STAGE

This is also referred to as overtraining. Here are the signs.

- A leveling off of your performance or an actual decrease in strength
- Chronic fatigue
- Loss of appetite
- Loss of weight and muscle
- Illness or infection, such as a chronic sore throat
- Injury
- Decreased motivation or lower self-confidence

Obviously, if you hit this stage, the party's over. Your body has gone from steady improvement to either no improvement or a backslide.

The problem doesn't always originate in the gym. You could be doing an excellent, well-balanced exercise routine with plenty of time built in for recovery between workouts, but other stresses in your life could be pushing you into overtraining. A few of the usual suspects are long work hours or friction with your boss; trouble with your wife, girlfriend, ex-wife, ex-girlfriend, children, parents, pets, and so on; and poor eating habits.

Good things can also create a level of stress that will push you into the exhaustion stage. Among these are a promotion that leads to new responsibilities; a new, exciting relationship; the birth of a child; a new home; and a damned fun nightlife that cuts into your sleep, relaxation, and recovery time.

## IMPROVING IN STAGES

You want to keep your body in the resistance stage for the biggest chunks of your workout time—stretches of 6 to 8 weeks are ideal, although a good workout program could go up to 12 weeks.

But from time to time, you have to return to the alarm stage. That is, you have to take on new challenges that mildly shock your body. Some guys never return to this stage after finding a program they're comfortable with, and that's fine . . . for them. You, on the other hand, want to keep making improvements. And improvements start with a shock to the system, from which you quickly recover.

## REACHING YOUR PEAK

The concept of peaking is usually used when talking about athletes who need to be at their absolute best for a single event (the Boston Marathon, for example) or series of events (the Olympics).

But from time to time, every guy has a moment when he wants to look his absolute best. Maybe it's a honeymoon on an exotic beach, a 10-year high school reunion, or the first day of pool season. That, too, is peaking.

Here's how to do it.

**Ab exercises:** In the Core Program, you did ab exercises three times a week. That's usually enough, although many guys do 4 or even 5 days a week before a major event involving shirt removal. If you do that, split your abdominal exercises into three groups—one for upper-ab exercises, one for lower abs, one for obliques—and rotate them in your workouts. The Index lists all of the exercises in the book according to which muscles they emphasize.

You'll still end up working all of your ab muscles almost every day, since it's physiologically impossible to keep your lower abs from contracting while you're working your upper abs, and your obliques tend to contract as a support muscle on all upper-ab and lower-ab movements. But at least you'll be doing different exercises each time you train.

**Aerobics:** Do steady, moderate-intensity aerobic workouts 4 days a week. On another 2 days, do interval workouts.

**Eating:** Cutting calories will bring out cuts in your muscles, but you have to do it intelligently. You're still trying to build muscle, so you don't want to cut any protein. Most models and body-builders cut carbohydrates way back or eliminate them entirely. You don't have to go that far, of course, but if there are some carbohydrate foods that you chronically overeat, stay away from them until you're past the event for which you're peaking.

## POSTPEAKING

Many guys mistakenly believe that they can stay in peak condition all the time. Unfortunately, the body doesn't work like that. Trying to keep it peaked for more than a week or two will lead to stage three, overtraining and burnout.

Instead, after you hit a peak, you need to take a transitional week or two off to give your body and mind a chance to relax, recuperate, and then prepare for another cycle of training consisting of a short alarm stage, a long resistance stage, and a peak of some sort.

What do you do during this transition? In some cases, the event for which you peaked determines your activity level. If you peaked for a honeymoon or vacation, your recreational activities serve as your transition stage—walking on the beach, sailing, playing golf or tennis.

If you peaked for a 1-day event that doesn't involve travel, you may struggle a little more with the transition. Your gym is right there, you're used to going there almost every day, and you're still excited about your workouts. It becomes a struggle to put the brakes on your program.

Failing to take a break would, of course, be a mistake. It may not catch up with you right away, but eventually you'd push your body past its limits and end up sick, hurt, or burned out.

Here's how to make a transition without changing your locale.

- Drop your formal program and play around with new machines or try new exercises.
- Don't keep track of your sets, repetitions, or weights.
- Do your favorite abdominal exercises instead of the ones from which you think you'll get the most benefit.
- Do your aerobic workouts at a comfortable, enjoyable pace. Let your mind wander. If you train outdoors, pick a new route based solely on the scenery. Don't track your miles or worry about your pace.
- Don't do any high-intensity techniques, like supersets in the weight room or interval aerobics.

## THE ULTIMATE BALANCING ACT

Many guys think that they'll fall behind when they ease off the throttle during a transition, but the opposite is true. The best athletes in the world train like this. They and their coaches know that fitness improves in planned cycles, not in a steady, upward progression. If you want the best body possible, you should train like the guys who know the most about training.

Of course, an athlete's peaking cycle is determined by scheduled competitive events, something a regular guy doesn't have. But we all follow the same calendar, and you can use it to plan peaks and transitions. Peak near a holiday, take a break to enjoy the holiday with family and friends, then ease into your next series of workouts after the transition.

You'll enjoy your workouts more and your life more. That's the balance that all of us strive for, but few of us hit.

Train hard. Train smart. Train consistently. And when it's time to ease off, let it go and have some fun.

# INDEX

Underscored page references indicate boxed text.
**Boldface** references indicate photographs.